Matron in Charge

Matron in Charge

The Life of a 1960s Nurse

EVELYN PRENTIS

EBURY
PRESS

7 9 10 8 6

Published in 2012 by Ebury Press, an imprint of Ebury Publishing
A Random House Group company
First published in Great Britain by
Hutchinson & Co (Publishers) Ltd in 1982

The Random House Group Limited Reg. No. 954009

Addresses for companies within the Random House Group can be found
at www.randomhouse.co.uk

A CIP catalogue record for this book is available
from the British Library

The Random House Group Limited supports The Forest Stewardship
Council (FSC®), the leading international forest certification
organisation. Our books carrying the FSC label are printed on FSC®
certified paper. FSC is the only forest certification scheme endorsed by
the leading environmental organisations, including Greenpeace.
Our paper procurement policy can be found at
www.randomhouse.co.uk/environment

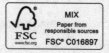

Printed in Great Britain by Clays Ltd, St Ives plc

ISBN 9780091941369

To buy books by your favourite authors and register for offers visit
www.randomhouse.co.uk

POST CORONARY BLUES

Ah, do not let me die in Spring
While soft winds stir the May-spiced scented air
While blackbirds pierce my heart with songs of praise
And bursting buds urge on the summer days.

Nor must I die in summer time
When roses spill their petals at my feet
When buddleia comes alive with fluttering wings
And bees make honeyed paths thro' moss green fairy wings.

And who would want to leave when Autumn's here
With cobweb mists and dew-wet mushroom patch
With browns and golds and ruddy chestnut glow
Autumn's no time for me to up and go.

So when the winter comes what then?
Shall I find rest beneath some scarlet-berried tree
Kept warm with snowy blanket, dark and deep
And wait for Spring to come and wake me from my sleep.

Part One

Chapter One

ONE OF THE first things I learned when I started my training a long time ago was that for many different reasons, some of them uncharitable, almost all nurses dislike nursing nurses. They like it even less if those they are being called upon to nurse come in on their own two feet, looking far too healthy to be taking up a hospital bed. Instead of being filled with compassion at the sight of a colleague hobbling into the ward, bearing up bravely in the face of a minor indisposition, they stand and watch coldly while she clutters up her locker with cigarettes and matches, tissues and paperbacks and other small comforts she will need until tests have been done to prove that there is nothing wrong with her and it was all in the mind as her seniors suspected from the start.

During her short and uneventful stay those dedicated to nursing the genuinely sick look pained when their colleague asks them to do things they are convinced she is able to do for herself. They do what they have to do grudgingly, leaving her in no doubt that they are neglecting more deserving cases for her. They make her bed in stony silence or talk to each other over her head as if she and they hadn't a thing in common. Life can be hard for a nurse who becomes a patient, whatever the state of her health.

Another lesson I learned in those bygone days was that nurses who go off sick with something not too serious seldom take kindly to the ministering angels whose mission in life is to get them back to work as quickly as possible. Nurses who imagine themselves more ill than they are resent being told by the night staff that according to the notes on their case sheet there is no earthly reason why they shouldn't be up with the lark every day, making their own bed and a few others in the ward as well, when they are quite sure that the mere effort of putting a foot to the ground will kill them. They take the greatest exception to being wakened at six or sooner, goaded into action by a trolley full of cups, teapots, milk and sugar left meaningfully at the foot of their bed by a tired night nurse. They mutter rude words as they grope for dressing gown and slippers to trail blearily round the ward, slopping in milk and shovelling in sugar, dispensing tea to patients who aren't always appreciative of the sacrifices made.

It is a foregone conclusion that after the last cup has been plonked on a locker only a few lukewarm dregs are left for the trolley pusher when she abandons it in the middle of the ward and stumbles back to bed. Such is the rigidity of hospital routine that she barely has time to snuggle down before a nurse, thermometer poised, prods her to life again. From then on throughout the day, meals, medications and other disturbances follow relentlessly, making it hard to catch up on lost sleep. I know about these things. I have been a patient and I have nursed nurses. I can speak with authority on both subjects.

I remember as if it were yesterday (though it was more than thirty years ago) being warned by my seniors that the patient they were leading with obsequious ceremony to the side ward was a nurse of very high rank who would demand the reverential treatment she was accustomed to getting from underlings like me. This, I was soon to discover, meant making absolutely certain that the bedpans I gave her were warmed to the correct temperature before I reverently eased her onto them, straightening her draw sheet so that she wouldn't even know it had been wrinkled, plumping up her pillows to the specified bulk and height and rushing with her dinners to the bedside before the gravy had time to set. Having a high ranking nurse in the side ward put a tremendous strain on the juniors and on anybody else who was summoned by the bell, which rang loud and clear and often.

Even the sister, normally so fearless, went pale when she heard that the patient on her way up from casualty was no less a personage than the matron of a rival hospital in a neighbouring town, admitted to us with a history of abdominal pain that had come on suddenly after she had eaten a hearty lunch with one of our local dignitaries. The sister's brow grew furrowed with the worry of knowing that the honour of our hospital rested on the way the alien matron was treated while she was a patient in one of our beds. A single sin committed by either a junior or a senior and it would be all round the rival hospital, and maybe mentioned in letters to the editor of a nursing journal, that we were an incompetent lot, lazy, good for nothing, a disgrace to our training school and a sad reflection on the sister's method of running her ward. So much hung on the smallest thing done for the very important patient that we were all a bundle of nerves by the time she went out, mercifully not too long after she was admitted, the abdominal pain proving to be no more than a very nasty tummy ache, which was as great a relief to us as it was to her.

The nurses were not the only ones who trembled at the thought of the lioness couchante in the side ward. Junior doctors and housemen called in to do a preliminary examination were nervously aware that the patient watching their every move probably knew more than they did about abdominal pain. They prodded and poked with far less confidence than if she had been an ordinary mortal, a nice motherly soul with a fondness for young men fresh out of medical school and still a bit hazy about the exact location of the stomach, especially one that is protected by several layers of solid flesh. They approached the flesh nervously, tapping at it in a half-hearted way instead of digging their thumbs in as they would have done under normal conditions. They gladly made way for the consultant when he arrived to take the burden off them and make the patient feel that she was at last getting the attention her high office entitled her to.

The consultant wasn't nervous. He was used to matrons. He had encountered many in the course of his career and was quite at home with them. He greeted the one in the side ward with the proper mixture of social and professional friendliness, then rubbed his hands together, not in an unctuous way but to warm them slightly before laying them on the well-rounded abdomen which the sister had discreetly exposed in preparation for his expert touch. He knew precisely where the stomach was and homed in on it without hesitation, both eyes shut and wearing the carried-away expression that consultants get when they reach their target.

Exposing a matron's abdomen called for considerable courage on the sister's part. A fraction too much or a fraction too little and her reputation would suffer the same damage as if she had been a junior giving a too hot or a too cold bedpan. Her fingers shook as she fumbled with the coverings. If the sister was off duty when the consultant did his round, whoever was next in line would turn back the bedclothes, lift the silken nightdress and reveal all or a considerable portion of the noble abdomen with the greatest trepidation, nerves stretched to breaking point.

The task had fallen to me once with another matron who had a different complaint and though by then I had passed my finals and was a staff nurse the responsibility so overwhelmed me that I uncovered quite the wrong portion and had to be reminded by the patient that she had chest trouble and not some gynaecological disorder. Rearranging the bedclothes and the silken nightdress under the chilling gaze of patient and surgeon had so discomfited me that in the end I left them to do it themselves while I went and fiddled with something that didn't need fiddling with at all. When the surgeon had washed his hands and gone I could tell by the look on the patient's face that should I ever be so foolish as to apply for a post at the hospital where she reigned supreme I wouldn't get beyond the mat in front of her desk. She had already rejected me as a probationer at the time when my mother was writing letters of application in my name to all the hospitals within reasonable distance of home. But since hers was a voluntary hospital and only paid probationers twelve pounds a year, my mother bore the rejection with fortitude and I did my training in a municipal hospital with a starting salary of eighteen pounds. This lowered me considerably in the eyes of our illustrious patient. Rumour had it that she never recovered from the shock of the National Health Service and retired an embittered woman.

The treatment meted out to matrons who became patients was exceptional. Nurses of less exalted rank were only accorded the same degree of reverence if they were admitted with something serious enough to cause widespread concern. The more junior they were and the fitter they looked when they climbed into bed, the less favoured they were by whoever was issuing them with bedpans, drinks and dinners, or slapping poultices on their wheezing chests or oozing sores.

Sick nurses learned to suffer in silence. If they so much as flinched when an ice-cold bedpan was pushed down their bed they were labelled at once as trouble-makers. If they dared to complain, however gently, that the poultice which had just been applied to their particular affliction was fetching the skin off in ribbons, they were accused of being fusspots with a laughably low pain threshold. If they lay quietly in their beds and didn't complain about anything, every nurse on the ward suspected that they were waiting for the right moment to start airing their grievances, the right moment undoubtedly being when the matron did the round one morning. Why else would they be submitting so meekly to chilly bedpans and red-hot poultices? No matter how hard a nurse worked at being a good patient or how impeccably she behaved, the cards were stacked against her from the moment it became known that she was a nurse.

I was a very junior probationer when I became a patient for the first time and neither the measles that put me off sick, nor the flourishing crop of carbuncles that followed the measles, were enough to cause anybody but myself the least concern. I was in trouble right from the very first spot. The sister responsible for the health and happiness of the probationers was beside herself with rage at having her nice clean sick bay contaminated by my measles. The carbuncles so incensed her that she ordered them to be poulticed and squeezed with such selfless devotion by nurses who disliked nursing nurses that I still bear the scars of the treatment I got. It was, perhaps, the memory of that first painful experience that kept me from going off sick for the rest of my training days, though being as strong as a horse might also have helped.

I was middle-aged and the matron of the Lodge before I had to steel myself for another stay in hospital. Being a matron instead of an unimportant junior I confidently expected at least a few privileges on the ward where I was to have a bit of minor surgery done. I didn't ask for much, just some nice warm bedpans, a few hot dinners and a side ward to enjoy them in. It was the thought of these little extras that raised my spirits when I was worrying about going into hospital.

The Lodge was a rather shabby collection of Victorian flatlets, administered by a charitable body and occupied by elderly ladies of limited means. Though I was happy to be its matron there was very little glory attached to the job. This was one of the reasons why I didn't get the side ward I'd been hoping for. Another thing that stood between me and my aspirations was that I was suffering from a complaint that nobody dies of, or so rarely that it causes quite a stir when it happens. One of the hard facts of hospital life is that there has to be some small element of risk in a case history before doctors and nurses show much interest. Charts that promise nothing but routine progress in the right direction rarely merit more than a quick glance and a few muttered words during the doctor's round. He and those following him have seen too much drama to be stirred by the trivial.

But in spite of the dullness of my complaint I went into hospital prepared for the worst. The residents had vied with each other to warn me of the terrible complications that would set in after even a most minor operation. I listened with only half an ear to oft-repeated stories about swabs, scalpels and scissors that couldn't be accounted for at the final checkup, making it necessary for stitches to be unpicked, a frenzied search made in the resulting cavity and a fresh lot of needlework done. This favourite fairy tale usually ended happily, with the missing articles being found in their rightful place and not inside the patient as had at first been feared. Though I didn't believe any of the stories I heard about wrong things being removed and things going missing at a crucial stage, I didn't look forward to having an operation.

Mrs Turgoose, one of the oldest residents at the

Lodge and quite the liveliest, had as usual been able to find a silver lining behind my darkish cloud. She had leered horribly and nudged me until I was black and blue while she dwelt with ghoulish glee on the possibility of the surgeon using me as a guinea pig and sending me back to the Lodge with one or two attachments that I hadn't had before. She was so taken up with the idea of my being turned into a bearded gentleman that I promised to give her a share in the fame (should such a thing happen) by seeing that she got her picture in the papers with double-spread accounts of how she had known me in the days when I was a woman. She dug me in the ribs again and went off to tell a few of her friends in the Darby and Joan club that with a bit of luck they would soon be getting a man as matron of the Lodge.

The joke had worn threadbare by the time she and other residents waved me off to the hospital. I remembered as I waved back that Mrs Turgoose had been the first to welcome me to the lattice windowed, white-washed building. She had bustled across the grass as I was standing on the forecourt, taking my first look round. After establishing that I was to be the new matron she had invited me into her flatlet for a cup of tea. Over the tea she had given me a short history of the residents, past and present. Now she was within a few years of catching up with her long-gone father. He, she told me often, would certainly have lived to be a hundred or more if he hadn't been a stubborn old mule and insisted on putting in his cabbages on his ninety-ninth birthday. He had keeled over as he was dibbling in the last spindly plant. Though Mrs Turgoose still remembered this with sadness, she said that it was highly appropriate that he should have ended his days in the cabbage patch. Considering that he had always spent more time in the garden than in the house, it was just the way he would have wanted to go.

The news that a matron was to be admitted to Female Surgery got there before me. Nobody had yet realized that being the matron of the Lodge wasn't quite the same as being the matron of a multi-storey hospital. Two student nurses were standing at the door, waiting to receive me from the hands of the porter and conduct me to a side ward. They unpacked my holdall, bought specially for the occasion, hung my new dressing gown behind the door, put my new slippers and my extra new nightie into the locker with my new sponge bag and arranged my tissues and paperbacks on top of the locker. I had already given up smoking so there were no cigarettes and matches for them to groan over later. After my personal effects had been dealt with they started on me. They helped me off with my clothes, on with my nightie and eased me into bed.

While all this was going on I noticed that though they were perhaps a little subdued by the idea that I was a high ranking nurse they were not as obsequious as they would have been under similar circumstances thirty years earlier. Student nurses aren't as easily impressed as probationers used to be.

I hadn't been in the side ward long enough to get a hot dinner when a rumour started to seep through the main ward that I wasn't a matron in the proper sense of the word. One of the patients had recognized me as I was being led past her bed. I heard later that she had burst a stitch by leaning out of bed to tell those within earshot, who passed it on to those who weren't, that her friend's granny had a flatlet in the Lodge and though I was the matron there it wasn't the same as being a proper matron like the one who walked round the ward every morning, asking people how they were and looking every inch the part in her crisp blue dress and lace-edged cap. The patient had gone on to say that as far as she could remember I never wore uniform. She was right, I didn't. Usually I flitted from flatlet to flatlet wearing a jumper and skirt, with added woollies in the winter. This, together with my greying hair and timeworn lace, gave me an unprofessional look which deceived visitors new to the Lodge into thinking that I was a resident instead of the matron.

The knowledgeable one had gone on to inform her rapt audience that I was only at the Lodge to be at hand in case one of the old ladies was taken suddenly ill, fell down and broke something, or was poorly enough to need nursing but didn't like the idea of going into hospital. She spoke nothing but the truth. She could have added that I stood in for home helps when none turned up, did a little plain cooking, invalid style, when meals on wheels weren't available, and was on call night and day to answer emergency bells. I also changed fuses, adjusted television sets and did numerous little repair jobs when the handyman wasn't around.

But, as I discovered to my shame, none of the things I did at the Lodge entitled me to a side ward. When the news that I was an imposter reached the sister's ears she had me out of it faster than I was put into it. She burst in the door, chest heaving and eyes flashing, and stood tapping her feet impatiently while I packed the bag that the student nurses had so recently unpacked for me. She steered me by the elbow past the patient who was responsible for my eviction, past the others who knew me for what I was, past the student nurses who had been deluded into thinking that I was a real matron, and to a bed halfway down the ward. It was a long and embarrassing journey.

It was plain from the sister's heaving bosom and the way the students were looking at me that I would have to work doubly hard at being a good patient to make up for giving everybody so much trouble when I was first admitted. I accepted their censure. Being of the profession myself I should have known better than to let them put me in a side ward. Common sense should have told me that times hadn't changed and such amenities were still reserved for very important people, or for those with complaints more dramatic than mine. It was a bad start to my stay in hospital and if it hadn't been for Dole I might not have enjoyed it as much as I did.

Chapter Two

DOLE WAS IN the bed on my left. She was fiftyish and plump. She had light blonde hair with very dark roots and wore see-through, low-cut nighties that made the most of her ample bosom and cut into the tops of her arms. She had a large vanity bag crammed with lipsticks, pansticks, mascara and rouge, all of which she applied heavily every morning after she had taken out her rollers and backcombed her hair. The only time I saw her minus her make-up was on the day she had her operation and the day after. She looked a different woman without it. Her friends called her Doll but the way she said it made it sound like Dole.

She politely looked the other way until the sister had flounced off, then she gave me a welcoming smile and at once began to fill me in with interesting facts about the patients, the sister and the nurses. I listened as closely as I could while I crammed things into the locker and arranged things on top. I got into bed very carefully, trying not to untuck it too much. I knew that nothing annoys nurses more than having their immaculately made beds looking as if they've been slept in. When I had wriggled my way down I smoothed the counterpane, adjusted a slight displacement of the top sheet and looked around.

In the bed on my right, propped up by a mountain of pillows, was a very old lady. I gave her a warm smile and a friendly nod; she glared furiously and turned her head away. This chilly reaction to the nod and smile discouraged me from repeating either too often. I beamed whenever I caught her eye, but the more I beamed the more she glared.

When I mentioned this to Dole she told me that the old lady behaved in the same way to everybody. She was even worse when her family came to see her. The moment they approached her bed she lay back on her pillows, eyes shut and lips pursed in a tight line, and refused to answer when any of them spoke to her. Consequently they only came on Sundays and cut their visit as short as possible. They were the last in and the first to go and didn't look back when they went through the ward door. I thought this seemed rather hard on the poor old thing but Dole said it served her right. You reap as you sow, said Dole, and if she'd been a bit more grateful for the things they'd done for her in the past they might have been doing more for her now. We exchanged a few more words on the subject, then I beamed and nodded at the old lady to let her know we hadn't been talking about her. As a token of good faith I offered her one of my fruit gums but she tossed her head and declined the offer without any thanks.

She didn't need a fruit gum anyway. Her locker was loaded with chocolates and fruit, brought in on Sundays by her family as a peace offering for not coming to see her more often. Being a chronic insomniac I lay awake far into the night and watched the old lady scrabbling among boxes and packages, selecting the goodies she liked and champing them with her toothless gums. The rustle of wrappers sometimes brought a nurse to her bedside but by the time she got there the wily old lady had her eyes shut and was giving a good impression of being fast asleep. During the day she lay back on her pillows and made feeble gestures to whoever was passing, indicating that she wanted a soft centre or a few skinned and de-pipped grapes popped into her mouth.

'Sly old cow,' said Dole one night when her sleeping tablet hadn't worked and she lay like me watching the chocolates being transferred from the locker into the old lady's mouth. 'Fancy her making out she's helpless during the day, then being able to sit up and stuff herself when she thinks nobody's watching.'

I leaned over and explained in a whisper that when I was a night nurse I had often seen patients who could hardly move during the day sit up and do the most extraordinary things in the middle of the night. Our sister tutor had given us a name for this but I had forgotten what it was so I made up another to give to Dole. She was greatly impressed by my profound knowledge of medical matters and in the morning she passed on the bit of false information to the lady on her left, who passed it on to the patient on the other side of her. So much was added during its journey round the ward that I hardly recognized it when it got back to me.

Dole was in with her back. She'd had it a long time, she said, and so far nobody had been able to get to the bottom of it. She'd had a great many other things that nobody had been able to get to the bottom of. Several times a day, before we had our operations and after we were over the worst, she leaned perilously across the narrow gulf that divided us and told me long and involved stories about the things she had suffered from over the years: things that had puzzled her GP, worried the consultants and finally had defeated the surgeons. Blood tests, urine tests, bowel tests and stomach tests had all been done to no avail. When one doctor insinuated that she wasn't as ill as she thought she was, Dole went to another to get his opinion. She went on worrying despite being told that there was nothing for her to worry about.

On top of all this she lived on her nerves. I was surprised to hear this since she was quite nicely rounded and ladies who live on their nerves are usually a bit on the thin side, not eating as much as they should and biting their nails instead. But Dole said it worked the other way with her. She only had to have a few words with her husband before he went off in the morning and it took a potful of tea and several slices of toast and marmalade to restore her equanimity and keep her going until she had her elevenses at ten o'clock. So instead of being thin she weighed fourteen stone, which bothered her doctors more than it bothered her.

The day before we had our operations a card saying 'Nil by Mouth' was hung above our beds. Poor Dole blanched when she saw it, rightly supposing that Nil by Mouth meant that nothing was to pass her lips for at least twenty-four hours. But when the worst was over the cards were removed and another was hung in the space above Dole's bed. This had the words 'Obesity Diet' emblazoned in large red letters. In accordance with its instruction she was given minuscule portions of sugar-free, fat-free and taste-free food while all around her were tucking into sugary, starchy things.

Friday was a bad day for Dole. On Fridays, those not on any special diet got fish and chips for lunch with steamed pudding and custard to follow. Dole propped herself up on one reddened elbow and devoured almost in one bite an inch of cod stripped of its batter, a rather large helping of a leafy vegetable and a puree of carrots. There weren't enough calories to fatten a fly. She had never been a lover of leafy vegetables, she said, but I persuaded her to choke them down so that she could truthfully say 'yes' when the nurse who took her temperature asked if her bowels were working properly.

Dole didn't like yoghurt either. The first time she was given a carton she stared at its contents, dug her spoon in and churned the yoghurt up and over and round and round. After she had tasted a bit on the end of her spoon she threw the carton down in disgust and called the nurse who had given it to her.

'I can't eat this, it's gone off,' she said, thrusting the carton under the nurse's nose.

'Of course it hasn't gone off,' said the nurse. 'That's how yoghurt always is. It's milk that's had something done to it to make it go like that.'

Dole stared at her. 'Well, I think it's a disgrace,' she said. 'I wouldn't eat sour milk at home so I don't see why I should be expected to eat it here. You'd have thought they'd have known better than to give you rubbish like that in hospital.'

The nurse took the yoghurt away and Dole sat and watched me making short work of the steamed pudding and custard which I hadn't had the strength to refuse in favour of something less fattening. Though I wasn't fourteen stone I had quite a few bulges and knew to a gram the amount of carbohydrates I could eat before waistbands started tightening. I read slimming magazines while I was eating the things they implored me never to touch, and I went on eating after I had doubled their recommended quantities. My little snacks were their main meals.

But in spite of the bulges I was still rather hurt when a young houseman had a bright idea one morning. He looked first at me, more than filling a chair in the day room, and then at the sister. Some silent communication passed between them and when I walked painfully back to bed there was a notice hanging above it with 'Obesity Diet' printed in large red letters. Thereafter I was given minute portions of low calorie food with cartons of plain yoghurt to follow. Dole steadfastly refused to look while I was eating the yoghurt; she said it turned her stomach just to look at it. But she was pleased at not having to watch me indulging in spotted dick every Friday.

I made a point of removing the red-lettered card when I was expecting visitors. The stigma of being on an obesity diet would have far outweighed the good their visits did. I could imagine the unkind things they'd be saying when they should have been listening to a stitch by stitch account of my operation.

Dole had, of course, heard the things that were said about my not being a proper matron and though she spent hours discussing her ailments with me and asking for professional advice, she rightfully regarded me as a patient with some specialized knowledge rather than as somebody who should have been unswervingly on the side of the hospital staff. She felt free to run down the sisters, criticize the nurses and tell me in the most outspoken terms what she thought of doctors who hurried away just when she had started talking to them about her back. And I, by then more a patient than a nurse, felt free to listen and occasionally add my own critical comments to hers. A lifetime of loyalty to those we were criticizing restrained me from agreeing too heartily with some of the things she said, while my reluctance to take up arms in their defence had its roots in the days when I was a wife and mother as well as a nurse. It was a cowardice I was often ashamed of.

During the early years when I was a part-time nurse, dividing my time between home and hospital, I used to get hot and angry when people who had been patients stopped me in the street and kept me standing while they bemoaned the fact that doctors and nurses were not as good as they used to be, and didn't behave like the ones on the telly. 'Emergency Ward 10' had just started to glamorize the best and draw veils over the worst aspects of hospital life. I listened, with aching feet and a fixed smile, while the lady in the paper shop told me that when she went in to have her veins done she was left on the lavatory for ages because the nurse who took her there had forgotten to bring her back. She could have been sitting there still, she said, if the woman in the next bed hadn't noticed she wasn't there and raised the alarm. The woman in the paper shop said she'd never forget it, her bottom was still raw with all that sitting.

I stood, still smiling fixedly, while the man in the supermarket kept me shivering in the frozen food area until he had told me that the young whippersnappers up at the hospital who called themselves doctors would have had his leg off like a shot when all he had gone there for was to let somebody look at his rupture.

The man, growing more belligerent by the moment, said that if they thought he was going to lose a leg just for the sake of a black spot that had appeared on one of his toes they had another think coming. The rupture was different, he said, he didn't fancy wearing a truss for the rest of his life and the sooner they did something about it the better. It was a crying disgrace, he said, and no more than you'd come to expect from this newfangled health service – it should be abolished and everybody made to pay for doctors and medicine as they'd done in the good old days. Hospitals would have to think twice then before they started messing round with people's legs, and for nothing more than a black spot the size of a sixpence.

The man in the supermarket and the woman in the paper shop told me other things aimed at destroying my faith in doctors and nurses. But I didn't argue. I knew that nothing I said would alter minds already made up. I knew also that it often takes a desperate situation to convince the sceptic that good occasionally comes out of evil. I hoped that the man with the black spot on his toe wouldn't have to lose a leg before he was convinced, but the next time I saw him at the checkout he had nothing but praise for the clever young doctors at the hospital who had so wisely taken it off before the black spot spread and did even greater damage.

I went from the supermarket deep in thought. I had watched men and women learning to walk again on their brand new shiny legs. It took courage to struggle up after toppling over time and time again. I had watched children as well, but then it was I who needed the courage. Having only one leg when your playmates have two can be a serious drawback when there is a ball being kicked around.

I hadn't been too disturbed by the paper shop lady's prolonged sit-down. Experience told me that there must have been a very good reason for it. Either there was an acute shortage of staff, a sudden emergency, or a simple misunderstanding between the nurse who took the patient to the lavatory and the one who should have brought her back to bed. Being left on the lavatory is a hazard patients face if they are unable to walk without aid. I was quite sure that whoever went to her rescue would have been full of remorse for the unfortunate incident and not short of hastily concocted excuses. The older the nurse, the more plausible her excuses would have been. Older nurses did their training in the days when whatever they did was wrong, so they kept a good stock of excuses to give to whoever caught them sinning. I know. I have used them all.

But for all my unspoken defence of doctors and nurses when others were running them down, I found plenty to complain about while I was in the bed next to Dole. Egged on by her I rose from my pillows in fury when the night staff clattered crockery or dropped something in the kitchen just as I was starting to shut out other ward noises and drift off to sleep. I glowered at the students who swept past me with their noses in the air when I begged them to bring me a bedpan, and I was quite short with a very young houseman who insisted that according to my notes I was suffering from something quite different from what I knew I'd got. We were at cross purposes for quite some time before he looked at the notes again and saw that they concerned somebody else. He thought it was funny but I wasn't amused.

'There, what did I tell you?' said Dole, who had listened agog to the exchange between the houseman and me. 'You can't trust any of them these days. It's a bloody good job you knew what was wrong with you. If you hadn't, he'd have had you down to the theatre whipping out something before you could say Jack Robinson.'

I nodded glumly. I was almost ready to believe her. I remembered the stories the residents of the Lodge had told me of similar mix-ups. Old Mrs Hunt had sworn – may she never move again – that when she went to have her tubes taken out she'd gone home with them all intact but without something else that she couldn't remember the name of. She'd had to go back later to have her tubes removed. The first time she told me the story, and even after several repeats, I wasn't convinced, but now I wasn't so sure that it hadn't been true. I was even less sure when I heard the patient whose notes had been mixed up with mine telling the patient next to her that she was having the lot taken out all in one go. I discovered that it was her teeth she was talking about, she had thirty-two and every one decayed, and I shuddered to think that it could have been me emerging toothless from the recovery room. My faith in doctors took a temporary setback, as did my faith in nurses.

'I bet things were different in your day,' said Dole, inciting me to mutiny after two student nurses who were supposed to be giving me a blanket bath let me and the water get cold while they talked over my head about the exciting things that happened to them at the student nurses' social club and at the parties they went to. There hadn't been such things as student nurses' social clubs when I did my training, nor did we go to parties. The ones we had in our bedrooms, with the light out in case the home sister came and caught us drinking lemonade, were strictly forbidden and very tame affairs compared to those which the student nurses were discussing. I was a little envious at the things we'd missed.

I was on the point of telling Dole that things were indeed different in my day when I thought about Pickering. She and I had often kept patients shivering while she told me about the exciting things that happened to her when one of her rich young men took her out in his Baby Austin. Pickering had a lot of rich young men with Baby Austins and some of the things she said they did in the back of them were almost as interesting as the things the students said they did at their parties. She would have fitted in nicely with the permissive age. She had the flair for it.

'And I bet you never kept patients waiting hours for a bedpan,' said Dole, puce-faced with waiting. Again I opened my mouth but thought better of it. In a flash I saw myself as a probationer, too busy polishing bed springs to want to drop everything and go to the rescue of a puce-faced patient. The matron was fussy about bed springs. She ran her fingers over them every day in search of dust. One speck and my future as a nurse would have been in jeopardy. Patients and bedpans took second place to gleaming bed springs.

'Things were different then,' said Dole, and I gave a Judas nod and scowled at a passing nurse. But even as I scowled I knew in my heart that things weren't so very different. Doctors were still dedicated to healing the sick, nurses were still nurses in spite of the hardships, and patients still rose from their pillows in fury when crockery was clanked and things went bump in the night. As I had done.

Dole and I were ready to go home on the same day. We were weighed before we went and to our surprise we had both put on a couple of pounds. We stared at the scales, convinced they were wrong, asked to be weighed again, then decided that the gain must have been because we hadn't stuck rigidly to the obesity diet. By removing the card when my visitors were due I could rely on them bringing in enough filling and fattening things to cancel out the cod stripped of its batter and the cartons of yoghurt. Dole had added her two pounds by a different method. She kept the card right side facing, but had explained to her visitors that 'Obesity Diet' meant living on bread and water and if they didn't want her to go home looking like a skeleton it was up to them to do something about it. Her husband, dreading that his buxom lady might be reduced to skin and bones, came laden with the gooey things he knew she loved. We had furtively swapped fresh cream slices for sticky jam doughnuts and little custard tarts for individual fruit pies. As was shown by the scales, the exchange had done neither of us any good.

In the manner of all patients who have become bosom friends during a short stay in hospital, Dole and I made great plans to visit each other and do wonderful things together when our convalescence was over and we were firmly back on our feet. But I never saw her again.

I saw her husband. He was riding past on his bicycle and when I called out to him he got off and waited for me to catch up. He told me that Dole was dead. When I asked him what she had died of he said he wasn't sure but as far as he could make out from what the doctors told him, it had been one of those complaints that nobody had been able to get to the bottom of. I said I was sorry and thought guiltily of how I, like the doctors, hadn't really believed she was as ill as she said she was.

I only saw him once after that. He was with a lady. She was fiftyish and plump. She had blonde hair that was dark brown at the roots and her lips were a vivid red. She wore a lot of panstick and her eyes looked as if they had been put in with sooty fingers. He introduced her as 'Beat' and when we shook hands I saw that she wore two wedding rings, one dull, the other shining bright. As they walked off arm in arm I thought of Dole. I knew she wouldn't have minded the brand new wedding ring. 'Good luck to them both,' she would have said, sinking her teeth into another cream bun. Heaven for her would be a place with lots of lovely things to eat and not a bathroom scale in sight. I had often dreamed of such a place myself.

When I was due to be discharged from hospital I had hoped that some kind, understanding doctor would come to my bedside, take my hand in his, and tell me how dangerous it would be for me to lift anything heavier than a duster for at least six weeks. This was the sort of thing doctors told patients when I was doing my training. But times had changed since then. Over the years the convalescing period had been slashed to the bone. When I asked the doctor who came to tell me I could go home how long it would be before I could go back to work, he didn't even take my hand in his. 'You can start next week if you want to,' he said.

I didn't want to. I had looked forward to a nice long holiday with his official consent. I hadn't had a nice long holiday for years.

After the doctor had gone I wrote a letter in a shaky hand to the charitable body that employed me. In it I said that it would be at least a fortnight before I recovered enough to lift anything heavier than a duster. They wrote back by return saying that in spite of the inconvenience it would cause, they supposed it would be in order for me to have two weeks' sick leave on top of the leave I had already had. They made it clear that they weren't too happy with me for being off sick, which quite ruined the next two weeks for me. I was filled with gloomy forebodings about the reception I'd get when I reported back for duty and it was almost a relief when the time was up and I repacked my holdall.

Chapter Three

I HAVE ALWAYS had a dread of going back to work
after being away, whether on holiday, on sick leave
or for any other reason, and I don't need a psychiatrist
to tell me why. The dread can be traced back to the
measles and carbuncles I had when I was a junior. The
reception the sister gave me when I reported back for
duty was chilly enough to be remembered for ever. It
was only a fraction more frigid than the greeting I got
from the nurses, who should have been overjoyed that
I had made such a splendid recovery. But there were no
fanfares to herald my return and no warm hugs to
make me feel wanted. Nobody was impressed when I
told them all I had endured since I saw them last, and
nobody stopped to look when I rolled up my sleeves
and showed them the scars caused by the squeezing
and poulticing. Most of the scars were on my arms;
those that were not I kept to myself.

The sister spared me a few minutes of her valuable

time to tell me what she thought of probationers who went off sick when the ward was busy and there were stretchers queuing at the door and extra beds being put up everywhere. At the end of the harangue she sent me to the sluice with instructions to scour everything in sight as penance for my sins. For the next few days she saw to it that I was up a ladder washing walls when I should have been having my meals, and polishing bath taps when I should have been going off duty. She had ways of dealing with juniors who pretended to be ill when there was work to be done. She was ably supported by the staff nurse, who shared her contempt for malingerers like me.

The nurses had ways that were just as effective of showing resentment at having been left with my share of work as well as their own while I was suffering in the sick bay. They haughtily excluded me from the little get-togethers they had in the bathroom when they should have been buckling down to some serious drudgery, and they included me reluctantly when they were illicitly eating behind the kitchen door when the sister's back was turned. I suffered as much from their cold shoulder as I had at the hands of the sick-bay staff.

Later, when I was a wife and mother as well as a nurse, there were more reasons for feeling uneasy at the thought of going back after being absent for a spell. Then there were children to keep me at home when I was expected at work. A shriek in the night or a more than usual reluctance to go to school in the morning, so long as I was sure there was a good enough reason for either, had me reaching for the phone to break the news that I wouldn't be on duty that day, or maybe even for a week or two, depending on the severity of whatever was keeping me away. The silence on the other end of the line while I was making my excuses told me more plainly than words that my absence would lead to the hospital closing down through shortage of staff. I came off the phone stricken with guilt at being the cause of such disruption.

There were few part-timers who didn't have children to keep them at home when they were desperately needed at work. It might have been expected that part-timers who were wives and mothers would have had every sympathy with other wives and mothers who went back to work weary with snatching their loved ones from the jaws of measles or a touch of flu, but such was not the case. Memories were short and nurses were human. Those who had been left to carry the load were themselves weary, and in no mood to offer their condolences. Like the nurses in my training days they ganged up against the one who had disrupted the ward with her absence and it was often a day or two before she was truly forgiven and allowed to participate fully in the gossipy meal breaks so much enjoyed by part-time nurses.

But if part-timers with children found life hard, so did the sisters who had to make out the duty list. They got headaches every Christmas and during the long school holidays trying to arrange shifts to suit everybody. None of this made them sweeter tempered when somebody rang to say that her child had mumps.

With my highly developed guilt complex about being absent from work, and my dread of going back, it wasn't surprising that I spent my convalescence worrying about resuming my duties as matron of the Lodge. At least there would be no irate sister waiting to greet me with a list of walls to be washed, taps to be polished and bedpans to scour, and no resentful nurses shunning me for doubling their work load. (Resentful nurses often exaggerate the pressures they are under while doing more than their fair share of work.) Instead, there would be a Lodgeful of elderly ladies, all in reduced circumstances, and all eager to bring me up to date with the things that had happened while I was away.

It was the little things that had kept me awake at night when I should have been enjoying my convalescence: silly little things that made me toss and turn, tormented by self-doubt. I had moments of panic when I thought of the matron who had deputized for me turning out perfect egg custards in the event of Miss May coming over queer when there were no home helps or meals on wheels available. My egg custards were never perfect. They either curdled through being overcooked or were still at the runny stage when I offered them to the ailing Miss May, and though she was the most gentle lady, and tearfully grateful for all that was done for her when she came over queer (which was often), even she had been known to mention, albeit in the mildest manner, that for a baked egg custard, or indeed any milk pudding, to have the necessary staying power it was vital that it should be cooked to a turn. Mine so often weren't.

Not only did my custards curdle but my semolinas went lumpy and had to be put through a sieve before they were fit to be served to a resident who was relying on me to produce the light diet that her doctor had prescribed. Neither did rice always behave the way the cookery books said it should. When it didn't I craftily disposed of the failure, opened a tin of pre-cooked rice pudding, heated it, scattered nutmeg over it and served it with as much panache as if it had been my own unaided effort.

I took care never to let the residents see me wielding a tin opener, it would have destroyed their faith in me as a cook. If the deputy matron's custards had never curdled, her chicken pieces had never shrunk and her fillets of plaice hadn't curled up at the edges I could be in for some adverse comments the next time I served an indifferently cooked invalid diet.

I had other faults which I feared might have been cruelly shown up in the light of the deputy matron's perfection. Though I tried to be a good listener when I did the rounds there were too many times when I offered an opinion that hadn't been asked for or got an argumentative word in edgeways instead of agreeing with whatever was said. I interrupted a long, long story with a little one of my own, forgot to laugh at the punch line or laughed when I should have looked sad. I wasn't always as patient as I might have been when an emergency bell took me with beating heart to Miss Coombe's flat, only to find when I got there that all she had rung for was to tell me that her little budgie had just piped his first word and she wanted me to be there when he piped his second. As budgies seldom talk to order, I was often halfway across the forecourt when the bell rang again.

I was occasionally less than honey-sweet when Miss May brought me from my bed in the middle of the night because she had wakened up feeling queer and needed a cup of something to send her off again. I was often ashamed of the things I said under my breath as I shivered back up my garden path after filling her hot-water bottles, finding another shawl to cocoon her in and plumping up her pillows which as fast as I plumped them collapsed in a mound of matted feathers. It was at times like this that I wondered whether I shouldn't be looking for a job that called for less angelic forbearance, a quality I was short of at two in the morning.

If the deputy matron hadn't offered an opinion that differed from anybody else's, hadn't uttered an argumentative word or cut a long story short, had laughed in all the right places and been full of angelic forbearance, I saw trouble looming. She could have endeared herself so much to the residents that I would have my work cut out to win them over again. It had been difficult enough to win some of them over when I first went to the Lodge; the thought of having to start all over again, especially with the difficult ones, was more than I could bear. I prayed that the deputy matron had had her little failings.

One of the most difficult had been Mrs Peters. From the day she moved in she had done all she could to make me feel like one of her own family. She had bullied me, browbeaten me, and blackmailed me into letting her do things that were strictly forbidden by the charitable body. Like her family I allowed myself to be bullied and browbeaten and had given up to her blackmail, fearing that if I didn't she would drop dead at my feet as she so often threatened. After each encounter with her I left her flat feeling a little older than when I went in. No matter how bravely I bore up under her onslaughts, or how meekly I gave in to her threats, I almost broke blood vessels trying to stay calm. There were days when I wanted to call her bluff to find out whether indeed she would have dropped dead on the spot if thwarted, but I never took the risk.

Over the years we had formed some sort of alliance, with her in control and me as the underdog. But the alliance was a fragile thing, hostilities never more than a slight misunderstanding away. If the deputy matron had been all that I wasn't I knew that Mrs Peters would be passing judgement against me for a long time to come.

Such were the problems that faced me when my sick leave was over and it was time for me to go back to the Lodge.

The deputy matron was waiting for me in the dark little house that was my official residence. I thought she looked tired. There were dark rings under her eyes, an expression of profound worry on her face, and a few grey hairs showing in the brown of her neatly permed hair. I couldn't remember seeing these when she took over from me the day I went into hospital.

She was wearing a navy blue dress with touches of lace here and there, black stockings and a pair of sensible shoes. From her breast pocket protruded a pen and matching pencil, and a thermometer case. Several badges were pinned above the pocket. She looked very efficient and almost every inch a matron. It seemed that my worst fears were about to be realized.

'Thank God you're back,' she said, ushering me into the matchbox sitting room where a fire burned brightly in the old-fashioned grate. My spirits rose a fraction. At least she hadn't enjoyed her temporary job so much that she resented my return. Perhaps, in spite of the navy blue dress and the important badges, she wasn't so very different from me. She went out and came back with a tray of tea and a tin of biscuits, then she sank into a sagging chair and kicked off her shoes. I saw that her ankles were swollen.

'Well, how's it been?' I asked her when I was settled in another sagging chair, drinking tea and thinking how nice it was to be home. She dunked a biscuit in her tea and sighed deeply. My spirits rose higher.

'It's been awful,' she said. 'You've no idea. It's been

one thing after another since the day you went. I honestly don't know how you cope with it all.' I smirked modestly and took another biscuit.

'It wouldn't have been so bad if they hadn't all gone down with the virus that was going around. They never stopped ringing their bells. I was rushing over there every minute of the day and night giving them antibiotics, cough mixture and everything else they wanted. I've never been so tired in my life, except of course when I first started my training and you know how tired we used to get then.'

We sat for a moment, recalling our training days, then I said how sorry I was that she had had the virus to contend with as well as everything else.

'It wasn't your fault,' she said kindly. 'You couldn't help being ill and you weren't to know there was going to be a bug going round. I wouldn't have minded so much if there'd been a few home helps or some meals on wheels but they caught it as well. I had to do invalid cookery on top of all the other things.'

Again I apologized for leaving her with so much to do. I realized that fate had played her a cruel trick in sending her the virus, when all she had expected was a quiet life and plenty of time to do her knitting. Her knitting bag lay on the sofa looking as if it hadn't been unzipped.

'How's Miss May?' I asked, after I had heard more of the horrors of the past few weeks.

The deputy matron smiled warmly. 'I should think she's the same as she's always been,' she said, dunking a digestive and fishing for the soggy bits. 'She didn't actually catch the bug but she stayed in bed to be on the safe side. She came over queer one night last week and she's been under the doctor ever since. I can't say I blame her. He's so dishy I wouldn't mind being under him myself, if you know what I mean.'

She gave me a mischievous look. I knew what she meant. Though I was a good bit older than Miss May's doctor I had occasionally cast an unmatronly eye on him when he strode into her flat, threw himself down on her bed and took her tiny hand in his large capable one. His bedside manner was irresistible to elderly ladies, and to middle-aged ones as well.

'I got ever so fond of her, but doesn't she need a lot of little meals when she comes over queer?' the deputy matron went on. 'She's so grateful for everything you do for her that I used to feel awful after I'd spoken a bit sharply to her when she got me up at two in the morning to give her some Bovril or fill her hot-water bottles. And I could never make baked egg custards the way she liked them. She said yours were always perfect. Mine weren't. They were either done too much or not enough. And I got into terrible trouble one day when she saw me opening a tin of rice pudding. I gather you always make them.' I kept quiet and thought about Miss May and her many little meals.

She had been a sickly infant, an ailing child and a delicate young woman. The doctor she was under on her fiftieth birthday had solemnly warned her that she wouldn't live to be fifty-one unless she took small nourishing meals at regular intervals. She had followed his advice and was now approaching eighty, as thin as a stick insect and as tough as a thread of silk. I sometimes rather naughtily wished that she didn't so slavishly obey her doctor's orders. Giving her nourishing little meals at three-hourly intervals was very wearing for me when she came over queer and couldn't cook for herself.

'And as for Mrs Turgoose,' said the deputy matron, 'I've never met anybody like her. She never says anything without giving it a double meaning, then she digs you in the ribs to let you know she's got to the dirty bit. She's a wicked old woman but I used to like talking to her. She told me things about the people round here that would have made their hair curl if they'd heard her. You should have heard the things she said about you. I didn't believe any of them, mind you, but it makes you think, doesn't it?'

She went off to fill the teapot again and by the time she came back I had decided not to ask her what Mrs Turgoose had said about me. I thought it better not to know.

'And how is Mrs Peters?' I asked, when another cup of tea had been poured. A haunted look came into her eyes. It was the look that everybody got when Mrs Peters's name was mentioned.

'Well, I might as well warn you,' she said, putting the teapot down with a defiant little thud. 'She's going to tell you some terrible things about me. I could never do anything right for her and she kept rubbing it in how wonderful you were and how glad she'd be when you got back. I can't think how you do it. Nobody could have tried harder than I did to keep on the right side of her but we were at loggerheads all the time. She got the virus, of course, and I had to strain her semolina before I gave it to her. She raved about yours. She said it was never lumpy.'

I felt a warm glow steal over me. It could have been from the fire but I knew that it stemmed partly from knowing that I wouldn't have to work too hard to get the residents back on my side.

The next morning I set out early to do the first round. I drank a great deal of tea and a fair amount of coffee while I listened to the different versions of the things that had happened while I wasn't there. Everybody seemed pleased to see me, even Mrs Peters.

'So you're back then, are you?' she said, surprising me by pulling out a chair and inviting me to sit down. 'I can't say I'm sorry. The one that was here while you were away was all right as far as she went but I didn't like the way she went round looking like a matron. It made me, for one, feel as if I was in some sort of home. At least you never look like a matron, which is something to be said in your favour.'

Her words restored some of the confidence I lost when they bundled me out of the side ward for not being a proper matron. I straightened my skirt, pulled down my jumper, and went on with the round, happy to be the matron of the Lodge.

Part Two

Chapter Four

WHEN I FIRST saw the gabled building where I was to work for many happy years it was as if I had found an oasis, a haven of peace far removed from the bustle of life, the screech of brakes and the smell of diesel oil not a stone's throw away where a busy road ran past the Lodge. Then I had stood and looked at gardens bright with flowers and watched fat pigeons strutting and cooing in sweet harmony. Foolishly I thought that nothing could disturb the peace that hung like a summer haze over red roofs and green lawns. But the peace was deceptive. I should have remembered that even Paradise wasn't all it seemed on the surface.

It hadn't taken me long to discover that if life behind the latticed windows, with their impenetrable Nottingham lace curtains (soon to be replaced with more modern nylon nets), wasn't lived at fever pitch, there was sometimes enough turmoil to splinter the peace and cause the pigeons to flutter in panic. There were days when high words echoed across the forecourt and strong language made the squeamish cover their ears.

One of my duties as matron of the Lodge was to see that the peace was kept, and to this end I rushed to intervene when one of the residents had a difference of opinion with another. I said soothing things, and over the years perfected the technique of siding with neither while giving the impression that I was in complete agreement with both. This required considerable skill in the art of diplomacy. The differences that arose would have escalated without my soothing words and conciliatory pats. As anybody who cares for the elderly knows, not every old lady is as sweet as the smile she flashes at the young policeman who sees her across a busy road. There were residents at the Lodge who would never have dreamed of turning the other cheek, even to the mildest provocation. They were the ones who had known so much hardship in their life that confrontation was preferable to retreat in the face of the enemy.

I was always very glad that the confrontations were confined to words and the occasional menacing gesture. There was never anything as sordid as a black eye or hair torn out by the roots, and the highest words and strongest language could usually be found in a respectable pocket dictionary or in the Bible. I should have been in a quandary if anything more serious had broken out.

Of all the small incidents that set neighbour against neighbour, two were guaranteed to bring out the fighting spirit in even the most placid resident. One was the hogging of the washing lines, the other the sound of a door being banged during the afternoon siesta. Either of these offences could turn a sweet old lady into a scold, and lead to emergency bells ringing out like carillons across the forecourt. It took only a very little bang at the wrong time to bring a resident who was good on her feet charging up my garden path demanding that I go forthwith and put a stop to the nuisance.

Miss Cromwell was very good at banging doors. She never had a siesta. She waited until her neighbours were nicely settled with their feet up and their eyes shut, then she put on her gaberdine coat and pork pie hat, slammed out of her door, took a short walk round the garden and slammed back in again. She took so many walks after lunch that there was often quite a little gathering on the verandah prepared to do battle. But she was a formidable lady. She towered above her opponents, making them think twice before they stood in her path hoping to dissuade her from banging her door again. The speeches they prepared were never delivered and I wilted when I should have been putting my foot down.

Miss Cromwell also hogged the washing lines. They were at the back of the building, well away from the public eye. No sooner had the residents filled them with billowing sheets and pillow cases, lacy little table-cloths and snowy towels, than Miss Cromwell stormed out of her door with a bag of pegs and an armful of outsize underwear. The tablecloths, towels and billowing bedding were pushed together at one end of the line to make room for her less delicate laundry.

She was the only one at the Lodge who hung her underwear on the line. The others were more modest. They had little collapsible clothes horses in their kitchens, where they dried the things they wouldn't have wanted the gardener or the handyman to see. Miss Cromwell didn't mind who saw her underwear. Even when she was wearing it she would sit on the seat at the end of the verandah, knees wide apart, letting everybody see what colour it was. Stew the handyman often passed remarks about her bloomers, but the gardener didn't. He was older than Stew and more of a gentleman. He courteously averted his eyes.

To me, Miss Cromwell's most irritating habit was

that of taking on the role of matron. If she was in when the emergency bell rang she put on her hat and coat and hurried to answer it. Since she lived in the Lodge and had no forecourt to cross, she was usually on the scene before I was. It took all my patience and a great deal of tact to convince her that it was my duty to deal with the crisis. When she was finally persuaded she would flounce off angrily, scattering residents to right and left and slamming her door with tremendous force.

Strangers to the Lodge were often confused by seeing two matrons when they had only expected one, and workmen went off scratching their heads in bewilderment after Miss Cromwell told them that the job they had come to do didn't need to be done after all. Scouts who came looking for jumble were delighted at being told by Miss Cromwell that they could have the fencing at the bottom of one of the gardens. They dug up the fence and loaded it onto their handcart, and were highly indignant when I rushed out and told them to put it back. They looked from me to Miss Cromwell and didn't know which to obey. She was dressed for the part so much better than I was.

Not all the battles round the Lodge were fought between residents. I was sometimes summoned to put an end to hostilities after an aged parent had turned what should have been a happy family gathering into a full-scale clan war. Here I had learned to tread warily. One word from me implying criticism of any of the contenders, all of the same blood, and they would be at my throat instead of at each other's.

Mrs Peters caused many a clan war in her little flat. A dutiful son, paying his weekly visit, got a heart-rending account of a daughter's selfless devotion compared to his own indifference, and the daughter had her indifference weighed so often against the son's selfless devotion that when brother and sister met they had nothing but hatred for each other. If they met under Mrs Peters's roof she sat on her beautiful antique love seat, content to let them fight it out and only putting in a word here and there when she thought the battle was losing momentum. If the sound of the squabble spilled out of the window, bells were rung for me and Mrs Turgoose came to her door, anxious not to miss anything if there was anything worth seeing. Usually all she saw was the family leaving.

Mrs Turgoose liked nothing better than to stand at her door listening to her neighbours arguing. Not of a quarrelsome disposition herself, she had the knack of leading a friendly chat into dangerous waters, stirring up strife with every word she said. When the battle had begun between those she was chatting with she would retire indoors, wondering how it was that women who had been bosom friends not ten minutes ago were now behaving like sworn enemies.

Mrs Turgoose's only sworn enemy had been Mrs Marsh, who died in the middle of one icy winter. But she had wept bitterly as she watched the procession that followed the warm-hearted Cockney woman she had so much despised. Mrs Turgoose despised all foreigners, and particularly Cockneys.

'I suppose she wasn't so bad, taking her all round,' she had sniffed, throwing a plastic arum lily in the funeral director's path as he walked with bowed head before the cortege. 'And I must admit the place won't be the same without her shuffling along the verandah in those disgusting plimsolls of hers, borrowing things. Though why she couldn't buy sugar and stuff like everybody else is more than I shall ever understand. Maybe it was because she came from London!' She burst into tears again and picked up the arum lily, which the funeral director had thoughtfully stepped over. Later she put it back in a vase with the other plastic lilies. Her flat was ablaze with plastic flowers which she kept in sparkling condition by washing them every Monday.

As a mark of respect for her old enemy Mrs

Turgoose bought half a dozen plastic daffodils and placed them on Mrs Marsh's grave, where they lent a touch of spring to the dark December days. Long after Mrs Marsh's relations had stopped putting real flowers on the grave, the plastic daffodils stood proudly erect and defiantly yellow, washed regularly by hail, rain and snow, and dried by the winds that swept over the cemetery.

'I never would have thought I'd have missed her so much,' said Mrs Turgoose on a morning much later, when we were having a cup of tea and remembering those who had gone from the Lodge since I went there. We had mentioned Miss Harrison who brought her piano in with her and died in the middle of the Hallelujah Chorus. We spoke of Mrs Beauchamp who had known better days and was convinced that our dear old gardener was the same dear old gardener who had tended her father's gardens when she was a girl. And we spoke of little Miss Lilian whose ginger cat had given me so many sleepless nights.

'Proper barmy them three was,' said Mrs Turgoose, grinning. 'But at least them and old Marsh had some life in them, which is more than you can say for most of them round here now. If it wasn't for Miss Cromwell slamming her door and Mrs Peters raising Cain with her family every week, we could all be living in a monastery where nobody opens their mouth unless they're praying. Though if you ask me, there's more goes on in places like that than just praying.' She gave me a painful dig in the ribs and leered suggestively. There was no doubt, she said, that monks and nuns had their weaknesses the same as anybody else. Good they may be but saints they most certainly were not. It was against human nature.

'But nuns live in convents,' I reminded her, 'they don't mix with the monks in monasteries so they couldn't possibly do the things you're accusing them of.'

'Where there's a will there's a way,' she said, leering again.

Soon after this a change came over the Lodge. Mrs Carter moved in to an upstairs flat and destroyed some of the hallowed hush which Mrs Turgoose found so little to her liking. Neither Mrs Peters's family squabbles nor Miss Cromwell's door banging could compete with the battle cries that issued from the upstairs window when it was thrown open to cool the room temperature.

Mrs Carter was a nice old lady. She was still quite active, did her own shopping, and went to church on Sundays. When she wasn't quarrelling she spoke in a soft voice with a hint of a Yorkshire accent. When she was, she shouted at the top of her voice and the accent was much more marked. She had never been even comfortably off and her tastes were very simple.

For everyday wear she had a small collection of pastel-coloured twin-sets which she knitted herself, needles clashing and flashing as balls of wool became jumpers and cardigans at an amazing rate. For going to church, and for wearing on not too special occasions, there was a rather dreary bottle-green dress and a matching bottle-green coat with a mock fur collar which hung in her wardrobe, protected from the moth by transparent plastic covers. For more formal occasions, and hardly ever worn, a dark blue dress and dark blue coat were protected by two more plastic covers.

On top of the wardrobe stood a large, round cardboard box. In it was her best hat, black and perfectly plain. This she wore with the dark green coat as well as the dark blue one. She did her shopping in a very old raincoat and a striped cap knitted with the odds and ends of wool left over from the twin-sets.

She was very thin. Her bust was almost flat, her stomach even flatter, and her hips were no more than a bony extension of her matchstick legs. Every year it was my duty as matron of the Lodge to run a tape measure round her lean form before she sent for a new pair of corsets from a mail order firm that specialized in garments for the fuller figure.

'Why do you wear them when you weigh no more than seven stone?' I asked her once, when I was jotting down her vital statistics.

'They keep my kidneys warm and hold my stockings up,' she replied, sealing down the envelope which the mail order form enclosed with its brochure. When the firm closed down through lack of support I had great difficulty in tracking down the type of foundation garment which Mrs Carter favoured. Eventually I found some in a small drapery store that had been taken over by a large Indian lady. She laughed when she unearthed the corsets. She didn't wear such things herself. She carried her weight proudly, letting the flesh find its own level under a magnificent sari. I envied her as I have always envied large ladies who don't go on diets and don't try to hide their largeness.

Once a month the vicar came to tea with Mrs Carter. She gave him little triangular sandwiches with the crusts cut off and a slice of seed cake. She made the cake herself and would sometimes give me a slice with a cup of tea when I did the round. I would have enjoyed it more if the seeds hadn't got stuck between my teeth. The vicar wore dentures that rose and fell when he laughed, and sometimes when he talked. If I happened to drop in while he was taking tea with Mrs Carter he was acutely embarrassed when he caught my eye while he was trying to dislodge a seed that had implanted itself under his upper or lower plate.

On Tuesdays Mrs Carter's sister came to tea. She too was a nice old lady, a year or two younger than Mrs Carter. Annie was short and stout with a pendulous double chin. Her heavy, florid face could have done without the two dabs of rouge that were carefully placed where the cheek bones should have been. But she was always expensively and immaculately dressed. From the time when the autumn leaves started tumbling down to the moment in May when clouts could be cast with impunity, Annie turned up every Tuesday wearing one of the many fur coats that must have cost a fortune in insurance premiums, and taken up a great deal of room in her wardrobe. Her twin-sets were of the finest cashmere and her dresses fitted to perfection her roly-poly figure. Her pearls were as genuine as the diamonds in her glittering brooch. She told the time from a jewel-encrusted watch. There was nothing about Annie to suggest that she was Mrs Carter's sister.

She had raven black hair which was newly set for every visit, and owed its colour and gloss to the regular and careful application of the correct lotions, mixed and matched by professionals. Not a wave nor a curl was ruffled.

Mrs Carter's hair lacked any such lustre. Once a rich auburn, as she told me later, it was now many shades of ginger except for a cottage-loaf structure piled on top which surprisingly had kept its colour. It looked rather conspicuous towering above the more faded strands. Mrs Carter's eyebrows and lashes had lost whatever colour they once had.

The two sisters were not on the best of terms. They had discovered at an early age that because they were sisters it didn't necessarily follow that they had to love each other. The relationship hadn't improved with time. After battling their way through to their middle years they could still find plenty to fight over now that they were nice old ladies, smiling sweetly at everybody but each other. It was this failure to see eye to eye which caused the Lodge to come alive on Tuesdays, letting the residents know that Annie had arrived.

As the friction mounted, insults flew out of the window and penetrated the walls that separated Mrs Carter's flat from those next to it. Mrs Turgoose threw a shawl round her shoulders and joined others on the verandah to catch as much as she could of the drama, and Miss Coombe, who kept herself to herself and did most of her talking to her budgerigar, put the cover on his cage in case he picked up any bad language, and peeped through her window to make sure that battle hadn't commenced on the verandah. She was a very nervous woman and got easily upset when the peace was breached, however slightly.

Even Miss Macintosh, who also kept herself to herself, opened her door a fraction and took note of some of the more shocking things she heard. Later, when she was passing them on to me, she shook her head sadly and said that if she had a sister to come for tea every Tuesday she was quite sure she wouldn't be quarrelling with her all the time. Nobody came to tea with Miss Macintosh, not even the vicar. She had kept herself far too much to herself.

It was usually left to Miss May to ring her emergency bell, dreading to think what two such nice old ladies could be doing to each other over triangular sandwiches and seed cake. Her flat adjoined Mrs Carter's and when I answered her emergency bell she wrung her hands in anguish and begged me to do what I could to restore order before the situation got out of control. It was often well out of control before I plucked up enough courage to knock on Mrs Carter's door and remind her of the rules she had promised to obey when she came to live at the Lodge. One of these was to the effect that the residents should at all times be of impeccable behaviour. I took this to mean that they shouldn't spend every Tuesday afternoon throwing insults around and disturbing the other residents.

The gentle rebuke that I dropped through the letterbox if the door remained shut was often lost in a fresh outburst of fury. If there was a temporary lull and my knocking got through to one of the sisters she would come to the door, ask me in, and invite me to referee the next round. This I refused to do. Once I had satisfied myself that grievous bodily harm hadn't been inflicted on either I gave them both one of my sterner looks, uttered a few stern words and left them, hoping that the words had sunk in. I knew too much about both parties to risk being their arbitress.

Mrs Carter hadn't been long at the Lodge before she gave me a list of her sister's shortcomings. Included were a number of character defects: selfishness, stubbornness, boastfulness and many more. Special reference was made to Annie's refusal to let others voice an opinion if it differed from hers and her infuriating habit of acquiring one rich husband after another. This, of all her failings, was the one her sister found the hardest to forgive. It was made more unforgivable by the undisputed fact that each of the husbands had left his widow considerably better off than she was when he married her. One by one they had shuffled off, leaving Annie to console herself with her collection of fur coats, a fine house on the common and a flourishing coal business which provided her with the wherewithal to go on a cruise in search of another rich husband whenever a decent time had elapsed since the last spouse passed on. Mrs Carter suffered keenly from her sister's successes, as she did from her failings.

'She's always been the same,' she said one evening after Annie had stormed off leaving the Lodge aquiver with her rage. 'She was quarrelsome from the cradle and as stubborn as a mule. And shameless as well. She had men running after her from the day she put her hair up. She didn't get those fur coats of hers for nothing, nor the swanky house on the common and that coal business of hers. It's wicked the way she marches in here every Tuesday throwing her weight about and bragging about all she's got. She'd never have any of it if she hadn't been brazen enough to go around setting her cap at men with money and talking them into marrying her. You can't tell me anything about Annie that I don't know.'

Marriage for Mrs Carter hadn't been nearly as rewarding. She had left it late to take the plunge and was a widow within a year. There was no fine house for her to boast about, no flourishing coal business and nothing left from her pension for luxury cruises. The only fur she had in her wardrobe was the narrow strip round the neck of her bottle-green coat and even that was only mock. All she had to comfort her in her declining years was a flatlet at the Lodge, the vicar once a month and her bad-tempered sister on Tuesdays. None of this was enough to put a lilt in her voice or a sparkle in her eye. She wore the look of a woman who feels that life hasn't treated her very fairly.

Annie's account of her sister's faults was equally comprehensive. She called in to see me after she'd had tea and a jolly good row with her sister. I listened as patiently to her as I had listened to Mrs Carter.

'The trouble with my sister, as you've probably noticed, is that she's got a nasty jealous streak,' she said, sitting down in my living room and opening her rather cumbersome coat. 'She was the same when we were little. She couldn't bear Father Christmas to put more in my stocking than he did in hers and she took toys off me and broke my dolls. Then, when we got older, it was boyfriends. She never had any herself and she grudged me mine. You're never going to believe it but she even tried taking my husbands off me. That was when they were alive, of course.' I tutted in a non-committal way and Annie took a small, expensive-looking vanity case from her handbag. She freshened up the two dabs of rouge, applied a fresh layer of powder and a smear of lipstick and looked complacently at herself in a tiny tortoiseshell mirror.

'She's nasty tempered as well,' she said, adjusting her pure silk scarf. 'She didn't speak to me for months after my third husband died and left me the coal business and the house on the common. Instead of being glad for me she was downright horrible. Thinking back, it was understandable, I suppose. She lived in one of those places that had to be pulled down when they built the motorway. It was a slum anyway, as I kept telling her, but she wouldn't listen. You'd have thought it was my fault when they moved her into one of those high-rise council flats on the other side of the town. I was always glad that you couldn't see them from the common where I live. Places like that tend to lower the tone, if you know what I mean.'

She was quiet for a moment, no doubt contemplating the horror of having the tone of the common lowered. Then she continued, 'It's a funny thing about my sister, she's never had what you could call a proper home. First there was the slum, then there was the high rise. I must say I've been luckier than her in that respect. But there, she'd never have been satisfied whatever she had. You can't help being what you are and my sister's never been easy to get on with. I expect her affliction's got something to do with it.'

I stared at Annie but she avoided my eye. Until then I hadn't known that Mrs Carter had an affliction. In spite of her spare frame and pale face she seemed healthy enough for her age. She had often told me that except for a bit of trouble with her bowels now and then she'd never had a proper illness in her life. I knew that her hearing was perfect and that she only wore spectacles for close work and reading. She had never needed a home help or a meal on a wheel, had never once rung her emergency bell and couldn't remember the last time she was under a doctor.

'What affliction has she got?' I asked Annie. She gave me a sly look.

'Why, hasn't she told you about it?' She sounded shocked. I said that there had been no mention made of an affliction on the medical papers which Mrs Carter filled in before she came to the Lodge, and she certainly hadn't gone into it with me.

'Well no,' said Annie giving me another sly look. 'Come to think about it, I don't suppose she would. It's not something you'd discuss with a stranger, which in a manner of speaking you are, no offence meant and none taken, I hope. She didn't even tell her own husband. He had to find out for himself after they were married and it came as such a shock that I don't mind telling you that we all thought it hastened his end. He didn't last long after that.'

I said that although Mrs Carter had told me she was a widow she had never spoken about her husband.

'She never does,' said Annie, knotting her scarf and buttoning up her coat. 'She married beneath her, of course, her getting on for forty and frightened of being left on the shelf. She wasn't like me, with men queuing up to marry her. But I wasn't afflicted like her.'

I knew it would have been easier to come to the point and ask straight out what the affliction was, but something stopped me. If Mrs Carter had wanted me to know she would have told me herself. None the less I was determined to get to the bottom of it in an indirect way.

'Did she have any treatment for it?' I asked Annie, hoping that if she did and I was told what it was I might get some clue to the nature of the affliction. I was denied the clue.

'She did,' replied Annie, 'but none of it worked. I remember Mother smothering her with everything when it first came on but it only got worse so in the end they told her she would have to learn to live with it. It ruined her life, of course, but as I used to tell her, all these things are sent to try us.' She went off in the taxi that came to collect her after the turbulent little tea parties, and I tried to think what the affliction could be.

The next morning I started the round early and planned it so that I would be at Mrs Carter's flat in time to share her nine o'clock cup of tea. She was an early riser and prided herself on having most of her housework done before the others round the Lodge were stirring. This caused strife among her neighbours who objected to being wakened at six by the noise she made when she raked out her ashes, clanked the dustbin lid and beat her mats against the outside wall. But she had risen early all her life. It was a habit she couldn't break.

When she opened her door I was greeted with the sweet scent of beeswax and lavender, with strong undercurrents of bleach and disinfectant. Mrs Carter's flat was polished to a high gloss and disinfected to a degree that made it impossible for a germ to live in comfort. She was haunted by the thought that at her age anything could happen and was determined that she would be prepared for it. With this constantly in mind she spent a disproportionate part of her life scouring, polishing, and looking under the bed for fluff.

She invited me in according to plan and offered me a cup of tea. I sat at her newly polished table and listened while she told me about the dozens of pairs of shoes that Annie had got in her wardrobe. As I listened I tried to get a close look at her without making it too obvious. I scanned her face for signs of pitting from an old skin disease. Except for a powdering of freckles her skin was flawless. I glanced at her hands, looking for warts, but her hands, though toilworn with housework, were without blemish.

When I had finished going over the parts I could see I dropped a teaspoon under the table. While bending down to retrieve it I tried to examine her legs in case the affliction was centred on them. But her stockings were not the see-through sort. They were dark grey and sturdy, designed to keep the heat in and the cold out.

Thwarted, I decided to try and solve the problem by a more direct method. Without any preamble I asked Mrs Carter if she had ever suffered from migraine or bilious attacks.

Mrs Carter looked surprised at the sudden switch to health problems when she had just launched into another attack on Annie. She replied that she hadn't had a headache in her life and the only time she had ever been bilious was when she took a trip across the sea from the pier at Eastbourne to Beachy Head lighthouse. It was the worst twenty minutes she'd ever endured. She'd vowed never to set foot on a boat again – and she had kept her vow.

Descending the anatomical scale I touched on appendicitis and the different manifestations of intestinal obstruction. After Mrs Carter had finished telling me about the awful time she'd had through eating an unripe apple many years ago, she went across to the dresser and came back with a large and very tattered book. It was a dictionary which dealt with diseases from A to Z, their signs and symptoms and methods of treating them. Some of the methods were strangely old-fashioned. Leeches were recommended for blood-letting, mustard plasters for congestion and Gregory Powder as a purgative. I knew about leeches. I had seen them in jars when I was doing my training and had learned how to sprinkle salt on their tails if they were reluctant to leave their prey when sated with blood. But I had never actually seen one in action.

Mrs Carter riffled through the pages of the book, occasionally stopping to show me the passage on 'Verminous head, treatment of', 'Stupes, belladonna and turpentine', and other fascinating excerpts.

'You don't need a doctor if you've got a book like this in the house,' she said, pausing while she concentrated on the common cold. There was half a page devoted to it. 'I never get a cold,' she said with justifiable pride. 'If I feel one coming on I do as the book says and dose myself with a drop of quinine in water.'

I took the book off her and opened it at 'Veins, varicose'. The method of treatment consisted mainly of avoiding wearing garters and keeping the bowels open. 'I suppose you've never had varicose veins either,' I said lightly.

'Never in my life,' she said. 'My legs are as milk-white today as they were when I was a girl, which is more than can be said for Annie's. You may not have noticed but the backs of hers are bulging. It's her weight that does it. She's always been fat and was having her veins tied when she was twenty. I know she's my sister and I shouldn't be talking about her like this but there are times when I feel downright ashamed of her, what with her weight and going round the way she does in summer without any stockings. She even paddles when she goes to the seaside. I've seen snaps she's had taken in those foreign places she can afford to go to every year. She makes a right spectacle of herself, and no mistake.'

I could imagine Annie paddling, lacquered hair staying put in the teeth of the stiffest breeze, skirt hitched high above bulging calves, her white summer handbag gripped tightly to stop it being carried away by the tide. I had watched women paddling, and had envied them from the depths of my sand-logged deck chair, too timid to do the same.

I pressed on, hoping that something I said might lead to a mention of Mrs Carter's affliction.

'You've got a lovely skin,' I said, gazing intently at her face. 'You must have been very good looking when you were young. Not that you aren't now but you know what I mean.' I came to an embarrassed halt. I knew what I meant but I wasn't sure if Mrs Carter would.

She sat very still, and I thought for a moment she had taken offence at my remark. Then she roused herself and glanced across at the huge mirror above the fireplace. The glance was involuntary, like the one that is thrown at a clock when time, past or present, is being talked about. Whatever she saw could only have been in her mind's eye; the mirror was too high to reflect her as she was. But she seemed satisfied with what she saw. She simpered modestly and ran her hands gently down her cheeks.

'Well, although I say it myself, I wasn't bad looking as a girl. I've always had a good skin, which is something that Annie's never had. And my nose is a better shape than hers. She was covered with spots from thirteen and she was in the front line when noses were given out. What with that and her running to fat it was a mystery to everybody how she was never without a man. I used to think it was because she didn't wear corsets. She wobbled all over the place, which is what men seem to like. And wearing no bust bodice made her wobble even more.'

I thanked her for the tea and left before the comparisons between her and her sister became too odious. I couldn't help wondering if a little wobbling in the right places might not have been more advantageous to her than being as thin as a rake and as flat as a pancake.

I felt very frustrated as I continued the round. The investigations into Mrs Carter's affliction had led me nowhere. It wasn't until much later that I discovered the nature of the thing that had blighted her life, and meanwhile I had other problems to solve.

Chapter Five

WE WERE FORTUNATE at the Lodge in that there were never any earth-shaking events nor hugely dramatic incidents. There was never a fire, except a very small one when Miss May forgot the little lamb chop she was grilling and let it burn to a cinder. She was so alarmed when she saw flames shooting from the grill pan that she took a dose of brandy before she rang her bell for me. The fire had fizzled out when I got there but Miss May was under her doctor for a week.

I never once had to risk life or limb rescuing old ladies from deadly peril. My duties as matron were mainly concerned with the more ordinary happenings; though being ordinary didn't make some of them any the less sad. There were the inevitable griefs when somebody who looked like living for ever slipped quietly and unexpectedly away, or put a foot wrong, either in her flat or in the street, and was taken to hospital and kept there.

When Mrs Judd put the kettle on one morning and was dead before it started to sing I felt guilty at being powerless to stop it happening. That she was putting the kettle on to make me a cup of tea seemed to add to the guilt. When somebody rang to tell me that Mrs Jackman's curtains weren't drawn when usually she was one of the first up in the morning, I was ashamed that I had slept through the night without anything warning me that she wasn't going to wake. As well as feeling shame and guilt, I felt very inadequate when these things happened.

There were other things that brought sadness to the Lodge. Mrs Smith's grandson died before he had time to get to grips with his O levels, and the verandah went quiet. Flowers were laid on his coffin and everybody wondered whether Mrs Smith's heart would ever mend. But the old can often find amazing reserves of strength to see them through such tragedies, and soon Mrs Smith could talk about her grandson without weeping, which she hadn't been able to do since they told her he was dying of leukaemia. Mrs Wilson's daughter died of a disease that her mother had been cured of years ago. Mrs Wilson never understood why she was spared while her daughter had to die.

Between the major tragedies, there were other, less painful crises for me to deal with. I was faced with finding a solution when little Mrs James in the corner complained that Miss Cromwell deliberately trampled on her garden when she went to the washing lines. Mrs Dean declared she had lost something of tremendous value and threatened to call in Scotland Yard unless the local constabulary sent in dogs to sniff out the thief, and Mrs Hunt, one of the oldest residents, who had lived happily upstairs since she came to the Lodge twenty years earlier, suddenly asked to be moved downstairs.

Mrs James was the only resident who had a garden. When she first came to the Lodge she had cried a lot and said she missed having a little plot to call her own. The old gardener, Herbert, who could hardly put one foot in front of the other so he had to ride a bike wherever he went, had taken pity on her. He cleared a small patch of nettles outside her back door, gave her some seedlings and plenty of advice on how to grow them, and was as happy as I was when she dried her tears. But Miss Cromwell disapproved of residents having gardens. She showed her disapproval by making a detour on her way to the washing lines and grinding the tender plants under her size ten heel. Mrs James, terrified of Miss Cromwell, put up with this for a long time, then begged me to assert my authority and save her petunias from a premature death.

Knowing how badly I had come off in previous confrontations with Miss Cromwell, I went to the workshop, where Stew the handyman sat reading science fiction when he wasn't in the mood for working. I ordered him sternly to do what he could to stop Miss Cromwell from upsetting Mrs James. He gave the matter some serious consideration and thought up the idea of chalking a warning on a piece of three-ply which he erected in Mrs James's garden. The warning said 'Keep Off By Order'. Miss Cromwell, not knowing who had issued the order and thinking it might have been the charitable body which was what she was expected to think, thereafter skirted the off-limit area. Mrs James thanked me for having spared her petunias and gave me a bunch of the self-set forget-me-nots which had appeared in her garden and were threatening to drive out everything else unless they were ruthlessly pruned. I didn't tell her that the warning notice had been Stew's idea. I basked in quite a bit of reflected glory while I was matron of the Lodge.

Mrs Dean's problem wasn't so easily solved. Nor could I turn to Stew for help, or even the old gardener. She was younger than most of the residents, able to join in the activities at the church she attended, and the events laid on by various organizations and the senior citizens' clubs. She had seemed perfectly sound in mind and body when she first came to the Lodge and I only discovered her little weakness when she rang her emergency bell just after I had left her flat one day. I hurried back, thinking she had been taken suddenly ill.

'It's gone,' she gasped, meeting me on the doorstep.

'What's gone?' I asked, leading her to a chair and sitting down beside her. She looked vaguely round the room.

'Somebody must have taken it while I was down at the dustbin,' she answered, wringing her hands in a despairing way.

I never discovered who had taken what while she was down at the dustbin, either then or on the numerous subsequent occasions when she was robbed of a priceless possession. When the obsession was at its worst she wrote letters to those responsible for administering the Lodge, and to the Chief of Police, accusing me, Stew, the old gardener, and the Methodist minister who called on her once a week of crimes ranging from grand larceny to petty theft. We were all under a cloud until she had found the missing object, and back under the cloud when she lost it again. I was under suspicion so often that I began to wonder if I was as guiltless as I knew I was. Imagined wrongs, like imagined illness, can affect others as well as the victim.

Mrs Hunt was ninety. Since before she was eighty I had been begging her to move into a downstairs flat as one became available, but she had vehemently refused, saying that no power on earth would persuade her to leave her dear little home on the upper floor. She went on refusing, even though she got breathless and had to cling to the banister on the rare occasions when she went downstairs. But suddenly she changed her mind. She rang her emergency bell and in a loud and angry voice demanded to know why I had insisted on her staying upstairs when all she had ever wanted since she came to the Lodge was a dear little home on the ground floor, with easy access to the washing lines and no stairs to climb when she had been to the shops. As she didn't do any washing, having several devoted daughters to do it for her, and hadn't been to the shops for years, her reasons for wanting to move were a little outdated.

Unfortunately she made the demand when there was no ground floor flat available and, failing a sudden unhappy event, no likelihood of there being one in the foreseeable future. When I told her this she flew into a rage and accused me of having no feelings for a poor old woman who had been pleading for years to be moved downstairs. Why, she fumed, should she be victimized and kept upstairs, when others, like Mrs Peters for example, could stroll along the verandah when she felt like it, have nice little chats with her neighbours, and take a bath whenever she wanted? It wasn't fair, she said, making rules for some and not for others.

I knew it would be useless to remind her that Mrs Peters never strolled along the verandah having nice little chats with her neighbours, and the only time Mrs Hunt had ever been to the bathroom was when she first arrived at the Lodge. She had done a tour of inspection, taken one look at the spiders that had come up the waste pipe of the stained, old-fashioned bath, and declared that no power on earth would ever persuade her to strip off in the godforsaken place. She had kept herself scrupulously clean with a daily wash in front of her fire.

After I had told her that I would do what I could to get her moved downstairs as quickly as possible she lit a cigarette and disappeared behind a cloud of smoke. She was a heavy smoker and had been for as long as she could remember. She didn't believe a word of the things they were starting to say about the habit being harmful. As God was her judge, she said, she'd never done nobody any harm and it was a bad job if at her age she couldn't please herself what she did. And as for smoking killing her, she'd never heard such rubbish.

She knew a lot of dead people who'd never had a cigarette in their lives, and she knew plenty like herself who smoked like a furnace and showed no signs of dropping dead. Everybody, she said, had to go some time, whether they smoked or not. Take her late husband for instance, God rest his soul, he'd never touched cigarettes but he drank himself to death before he was forty and left her with a houseful of children to bring up on what she got from the Assistance Board and by taking in washing. She drew furiously on her cigarette while she was telling me this. Despite her pious prayer for her husband's soul she had never forgiven him for shirking his responsibilities by dying at forty.

I waited until she had stopped coughing, then I made a suggestion that wasn't well received.

'Why don't you give it up? Then maybe you wouldn't cough so much.' I had only recently given it up myself and was feeling virtuous though sadly deprived. It hadn't been easy for me.

'You'll never do it,' said Stew, who had little faith in smokers trying to stop smoking. 'My dad tried it once but his piles got so bad that he had to have a fag to keep his mind off them.' Stew's dad had been a gravedigger until he retired. The piles were a legacy from sitting on cold slabs while he ate his lunch.

'I gave it up and I'm sure you could if you tried. Think of all the money you'd save.'

Mrs Hunt lit another cigarette from the smouldering end of her previous one and I looked away. Though I had managed to make Stew eat his words, and had amazed family and friends who were so sure I wouldn't be able to give it up that they kept offering me cigarettes to test my will power, I still had the urge to rush out and buy a packet of my favourite brand when I saw somebody take the first satisfying puff.

'I don't want to stop coughing and what's the use of me saving money?' she said, letting the smoke trickle down her nose in a tantalizing way. 'It's my only bit of pleasure and I can see no sense in going without fags to keep my family in luxury after I've gone. There's enough put aside to bury me with and that's all that matters at my age.' I gave up trying to convert her. I could offer her no alternative pleasure, and remembering how dreary my life had been when I first stopped smoking I wasn't sure that it would be the right thing for her.

Finding a ground floor flat for Mrs Hunt wasn't in the end as difficult as I had thought it would be, but at first the problem seemed insoluble. Since there wasn't one available I would have to find a volunteer to move up and let her come down. The thought gave me restless nights. Those on the ground floor, with easy access to the washing lines, no stairs to climb when they came back from doing their shopping, and a front as well as a back door to pop out of if they wanted a chat or a breath of fresh air, wouldn't want to exchange for something less commodious, even to benefit Mrs Hunt. I approached Mrs James with the proposition that she should move upstairs. She was young enough to do the things she wanted to do without getting breathless. She shifted uneasily in her chair, blew her nose and wiped her glasses, then screwed up courage to refuse my request.

'I shouldn't like you to think I was selfish or anything like that, but it's the garden, you see. I've just got it looking nice and Bert's promised to give me some bedding plants out of his greenhouse. I couldn't look after them properly if I went upstairs.'

Bert was the old gardener. In return for keeping Mrs James supplied with bedding plants he occasionally shared her evening meal. Though a bachelor and used to cooking for himself he wasn't above propping his bike up outside her back door and sampling hers for a change, and she, a widow, was happy to have a man to cook for so long as he didn't outstay his welcome or demand more than a substantial helping of steak and kidney pie in return for his kindness. Herbert's feet would never have got him up the stairs, so moving Mrs James would have ruined both her pleasure in the garden and a beautiful friendship. I patted her hand and told her not to worry, I would be sure to think of something soon.

I didn't mention the matter to Miss May. Though she hardly ever ventured out, and then only after a great deal of preparation and some guidance on putting one foot in front of the other, she needed a lot of attention when she came over queer. Even when she hadn't quite come over queer she was usually just on the verge. Having to run up a flight of stairs to give her three-hourly meals, and several times in between when she wanted a cup of something to stay her, would have added considerably to my work load. But she had such a kind heart that if she'd known the predicament I was in she would have drowned me in tears and murmured pitifully that it would be better for everybody if she 'went' and left her flat vacant for dear Mrs Hunt. It would have taken me all morning to persuade her that she mustn't think of 'going'.

I didn't waste time trying to pressurize Mrs Peters into volunteering. Though she had twice blackmailed me and her doctors into getting permission for her to move from one flat to the other and back again (strictly forbidden unless there was some excellent reason for it, which in Mrs Peters's case there wasn't) she was the last person in the world to offer to move for somebody else's good. But in fairness to her I knew that even if her breathing wasn't as bad as she pretended when she wanted to get her own way, her family had told me that when she was staying with them it took three of them to manoeuvre her up and down the stairs every time she went to the lavatory. I couldn't see Stew and the old gardener wanting to drop everything and come to my aid if she got stuck climbing up to her flat after a trip to the supermarket.

Finally I thought of Miss Coombe. She was still fairly spry and could manage stairs so long as there was a rail for her to cling to. She was also very kind hearted and would do all in her power to help anybody, despite her shyness.

'I'm worried about Mrs Hunt,' I said, after another night of tossing and turning, picturing Mrs Hunt tumbling downstairs and landing in a crumpled heap. Miss Coombe turned from the opulent cage that housed her latest budgerigar. The cage was fully furnished. The living space was cluttered with little ladders, tiny tinkling bells, swinging mirrors, cuttle-bones, iodine blocks and long golden millet sprays. The floor was close carpeted with a sand sheet, changed every morning for another of a similar pattern.

'Is she ill?' she asked anxiously.

'No, not exactly ill,' I said, 'but she's suddenly decided that she wants to come downstairs and I haven't anywhere to put her. I need somebody to change flats with her.'

Miss Coombe passed on the information to the budgie, whose name was Suzie. The two previous occupants of the chromium cage were Billy and Joey. Billy had been eaten by a ginger cat that made an illegal entry into the Lodge; Joey spread his wings one day and flew out of a window which Miss Coombe had carelessly forgotten to close before she released him for his afternoon flutter round the flat. Though the latest arrival was indisputably male, Miss Coombe had decided to call him Suzie, hoping to sever the chain of misfortune that had robbed her of Billy and Joey.

Compared with his predecessors Suzie lived a very dull life. Both Billy and Joey had been wizards at football from an early age, skilfully dribbling a miniature plastic ball through plastic goal posts, enthusiastically applauded by their besotted mistress after each goal was scored. But Suzie was cosseted. Instead of being given his freedom two or three times a day to play ball games, or to flit from pieces of bric-a-brac to objets d'art, Suzie stayed behind bars, desultorily pecking at the things that littered his cage, or gazing at himself in a mirror. On the rare occasions when he was allowed out he drove Miss Coombe frantic by disappearing up the chimney and coming down streaked with soot. Neither Billy nor Joey had ever done such a thing.

On top of his other handicaps, poor Suzie was backward in talking. Unlike the others, who could reel off whole sentences by the time they were two, he was getting on for three before he could say his name. The young vet who was frequently called in to check on the little bird's health had gravely opined that the reason why Suzie wouldn't say Suzie was that he knew he was a boy and having a girl's name did terrible things to his ego. Miss Coombe was so upset by this that she promptly rechristened him Danny, but no sooner had she done so than he gave a faint squeak that sounded like Suzie and she changed it back again. But the vet had been right. Irreparable damage had been done. When at last he started to talk he had a pronounced lisp: he also developed a rather peculiar walk and spent a lot of his time in front of a mirror preening his feathers.

Miss Coombe relied a lot on her budgerigars for companionship. She had few friends, being of a retiring nature, and only one surviving relative. She had applied for a flatlet in the Lodge after the last family she kept house for broke the news that her days as their housekeeper were numbered. They were having an au pair girl from Sweden to take her place. Miss Coombe had never heard of au pair girls from Sweden and didn't know what to expect. When the beautiful young lady arrived she looked her up and down, took in the shining, waist-length hair, the long, long legs and the hands that had never touched a pan scrubber, and wondered how anybody who looked so much like a film star would cope with the thousand and one things which Miss Coombe had been doing for the family since the first of their four young children was born.

She had packed her bags, tearfully kissed the children and gone to live with her cousin in Dorset. There she had stayed until she got a letter from the selection committee of the charitable body, saying that as she was clean, sober, provident, and a resident of the town by virtue of having been employed there for several years, she filled all the requirements necessary for being granted a flatlet and could move in at her earliest convenience. With some of the money she had saved by being sober and provident she bought one or two pieces of good second-hand furniture, a few bits of nice china, a busy Lizzie in a clay pot and a budgerigar in a chromium cage. Then she moved in. It was the first time in her life that she had had a home of her own.

An orphan from infancy, she had gone from institution to institution until at fourteen she was sent out to service. Over the years she had kept house for a succession of doctors with small incomes and large families. She had faithfully scrubbed their floors, beaten their carpets, cooked their meals and done their washing. Between all this she had taken charge of each new baby as it arrived, and the not so new ones as well. In those days, said Miss Coombe, things were different. No sooner was the mother able to brave the nursery than she was in an interesting condition again and had to spend most of the day sitting with her feet up, drinking endless cups of weak beef tea.

'It must have been terribly tiring, having all the housework to do as well as looking after the children,' I said, when Miss Coombe was telling me about a doctor she worked for once who had six very young children and an ailing wife.

She sat for a moment, seeing it all in the fire. The flames leaped up the chimney and the log that the church had sent with her Christmas parcel sizzled damply. I had gone across to tell her that the vet would be coming in the morning to trim Billy's claws and beak. (Billy hadn't yet been eaten by the ginger cat.) She had invited me in, made a cup of tea and I was listening while she reminisced.

'Yes, I used to get tired,' she said. 'But there were compensations. I was a strong young woman and I dearly loved the children. Mondays were the worst. I had to be up at four to start the washing and get the first lot of whites in the copper before the children were down clamouring for their breakfasts. Washing was hard work then. We didn't have machines like they do today. Things had to be rubbed and boiled and put through the mangle. I hated mangling. They were heavy old iron things that took all your strength to turn.'

I knew about heavy iron mangles. We'd had one at home when I was a girl. It clanked and rumbled while it was squeezing the water out of the washing and it was as much as my mother could do to turn it. There had been mangles brought to the Lodge by newcomers who didn't want to part with their faithful washday friend, but the kitchens were small, too small to house such monsters, and the heritable body refused to have them cluttering up the environment. Wistful glances followed the scrap metal merchants who came to take them away. Losing a mangle was like losing a link with a bygone age.

Some of the residents bought, or had bought for them, one of the little table contraptions that either fell off in the middle of devouring a towel or clamped its jaws together and obstinately refused a folded sheet. Others turned to the bagwash. A man called once a week, collected the dirty washing and brought it back, fairly clean but still very damp, stuffed in a calico bag. This left creases that were hard to get out, even with the flat irons which most of the residents still used.

Mrs Peters would have neither the bagwash nor the little table contraption. She clung to her mangle. She kept it outside her back door, covered with an old patchwork quilt. Visiting committees commented on it when they did their tours of inspection but nobody dared to challenge Mrs Peters. The mangle stayed where it was until Mrs Peters could no longer turn the handle. When her daughters started doing her washing, and getting into terrible trouble for the way they did it, one of her sons came and trundled the mangle away on a handcart. She never knew it had gone.

An odd note came into Miss Coombe's voice when she was telling me how kind the doctor with the six children and the invalid wife was to her while she was slaving over the kitchen range and the wash boiler for little more than her keep.

'I'd never have stayed if it hadn't been for him,' she said, gazing steadfastly into the fire. 'He was so wonderfully kind and treated me as if I'd been one of the family instead of his housekeeper. But with six children and a delicate wife he needed somebody like me to take care of things. I stayed for a year or two after she died, then he got married again and his new wife took over. I started feeling pushed out so I left.'

I couldn't help wondering how hurt she had been, and how pushed out she felt, when the new young wife took over. I had heard similar stories from other spinster ladies at the Lodge. Even Miss May sighed deeply when she told me about the young curate who came to the house regularly to comfort her after her sister died, but who, she discovered, was married. Miss Coombe wasn't the only one who had once dreamed dreams.

When I had finished telling Miss Coombe about the problems I was having with Mrs Hunt she went over to the mantelpiece and fetched a letter that had been propped behind the clock. It was already crumpled with being read so often. She didn't get many letters and any she got provided her with reading matter until the next one came. When she had read them so often that she knew them off by heart she put them in an old biscuit tin with other letters that she had kept since the First World War. As well as the letters there were faded pictures. One of these was of a young woman seated at a table, staring into the depths of an aspidistra. Miss Coombe thought it might be a photograph of her mother, though she could never be sure. It had been given to her when she left the workhouse to go into service but nobody ever told her who it was. I said there was little doubt that it was her mother because she had dimples in her cheeks and so had Miss Coombe. But Miss Coombe laughed and said her dimples had turned into wrinkles long ago.

The letter she showed me was from the cousin in Dorset. It was a cry for help. She had been recently widowed and desperately needed a companion to make her life less empty than it had been since her husband died. She pleaded with Miss Coombe to consider leaving the Lodge to go and live with her.

'I shall go, of course,' said Miss Coombe firmly. 'She's the only relative I've got. I couldn't possibly stay here when she needs me so badly. Her husband was always so kind to me and they made me more than welcome when I stayed there before I came to live here.' I saw there would be no point in trying to make her alter her decision.

Miss Coombe was a gentle lady with a mind of her own. It seemed sad that she should be giving up the home she had waited so long to get, but I understood her reasons. She had spent her life rendering devoted service to others; she would see it as her duty to go on doing so for as long as she was needed.

'How old is your cousin?' I asked her. She smiled, catching the drift of my thoughts.

'It depends on what you mean by old. She's a year or two older than me but by no means senile. She was fortunate enough to marry a man who did all he could to spoil her. But she was never spoiled. Unlike some women who have lost devoted husbands, she is quite capable of looking after herself, and me as well if necessary. But as you can see from her letter she misses the companionship and as we get on very well together it was only natural that she should turn to me. We shall manage nicely so you don't need to worry.' She put the letter back into the envelope and went to tell Suzie that they would shortly be going to live with their cousin in Dorset. Suzie showed a marked lack of interest.

I was reassured to hear that Miss Coombe's cousin hadn't been too much affected by having an adoring husband. There were those at the Lodge who would never recover from losing loved ones who had antici-pated their every want. Mrs Payne wept every morning as she spread butter and marmalade on her toast. She choked over the tea she had poured out for herself, recalling happier times when her husband had done it all for her. He had smoothed her path so lovingly that she was unutterably lost without him. Mrs Baker, who wasn't with us long, had spent her last few months waiting for the time when she would take the same winding road to the crematorium that her husband had taken, and poor Mrs Eaves would be haunted to the end of her days by the thought that she wasn't with her man when he died. She had come back from visiting a friend, expecting her husband to be at the door to greet her as he always did, but he was sitting in his chair exactly as when she left him, except that he was dead.

I was sorry to see Miss Coombe go from the Lodge. She and her budgies had given me a great deal of happiness as well as sadness. I had mourned with her when Billy got eaten, and had even wept a little when Joey took to his wings and was never seen again. I had cooed over new arrivals and rejoiced when they mastered 'Who's a pretty boy then?' I had been grateful to them all for bringing joy to their gentle mistress.

Suzie was Miss Coombe's chief concern while she was preparing to leave. Her cousin had a cat. Through an exchange of letters it had been established that the cat was fat and lazy and unlikely to take any action against Suzie. But Miss Coombe still worried. She lay awake at night wondering how big a risk there was of her budgie being eaten. In the weeks before she went she paced to and from the cage impressing upon him the importance of keeping clear of pussies' claws. He paid no heed to her warnings and went on preening himself as if there were no such things as cats. I hoped for both their sakes that he wouldn't have to learn the hard way.

When the hired car containing Miss Coombe and Suzie had disappeared round the corner I looked for Stew to tell him that the downstairs flat was empty and he must get it ready as quickly as possible for Mrs Hunt. Despite an accumulation of unfinished jobs he was in his workshop reading science fiction. I gave him a sharp look to show my displeasure but he turned over another page and went on reading. Like Suzie, he could be very unheeding sometimes.

Chapter Six

WHEN STEW FIRST came to the Lodge, not long after I arrived, he was a shy young man, plagued with acne and given to turning bright red at the least little thing. He would back out hastily when he went to one of the flatlets to tack down a carpet or put a washer on a tap and the door was opened by an old lady with next to nothing on. Even after I explained that she had merely had a lapse of memory and forgotten to dress herself properly, he still hung back. I had to speak to him sternly before he would agree to going in and doing the job he had been sent there to do. He insisted that I went in with him. I wasted a great deal of time trying to keep Miss Harrison covered while Stew fixed something that had fallen apart. Things were always falling apart at the Lodge and Miss Harrison had frequent lapses when she forgot to put on anything except a vest.

As well as being embarrassed by near-naked ladies,

Stew was reluctant to listen when the residents were eager to talk, and not as impressed as he might have been when they told him stories of how things were when they were young.

'That woman in number sixteen kept me there for hours talking about the days when there weren't any cars on the streets but only horses and carts,' he said one morning when he was making excuses for not sweeping up the leaves on the forecourt.

'Well, you should have known there were only horses and carts when she was young. Cars didn't start until later.' As I wasn't sure when they started I didn't set a precise date.

'I know all about that,' he said. 'But she says things were better then without petrol and stuff polluting the air. I felt like telling her that if it came to the push I'd rather be polluted with a drop of petrol than a load of horse manure. The streets must have looked disgusting and ponged something awful, especially if the council men were out on strike.' He had just bought his first Morris Minor on hire purchase and was busily rounding up girls to test the springs in the back seat. They wouldn't have had nearly as much fun at the back of a horse.

Over the years he had conquered his shyness, lost his spots, and didn't turn a hair when he walked into a flatlet and was greeted by a lady dressed only in a vest. He cultivated a taste for tea that almost matched his taste for beer while he listened attentively to whatever anybody cared to tell him, only occasionally interrupting to nod sagely and agree with whatever was said. I sometimes suspected that he spent a lot of his time listening when he should have been working, but if I suggested this to him he gave me a hurt look and reminded me of the number of times I'd told him off for not listening, and scuttling away when the residents wanted to talk, as if afraid that they were going to bite him. It would have been no use pointing out that I only did that when he first came to the Lodge and was too scared to open his mouth. Stew had an answer for everything when he found his tongue and got rid of his acne.

Once he had lost his shyness he was as good as another pair of hands to me. He managed to persuade Miss Cromwell that she wasn't the matron, though she still had days when she knew she was. He calmed Mrs Dean with a word when she was running round in circles looking for things she hadn't lost, and he wasn't above answering an emergency bell if he knew I was busy answering another. He would even help me to lift somebody out of the bath when she was heard shouting that she was stuck.

'Ups-a-daisy, steady old girl,' he cried enthusiastically as we heaved an amply built lady up the slippery slopes of the prehistoric bath. He was always punctilious about shutting his eyes while we did the heaving, and kept them shut until I told him it was safe to open them. This respect for their modesty meant that the amply built never minded him giving me a hand when they got stuck, especially as the alternative was to stay stuck until assistance arrived in the shape of a home help or a meals-on-wheels lady. The old gardener didn't volunteer for the task. He was afraid of getting lumbago.

Taking a bath at the Lodge wasn't the bubbly, luxurious, soaking experience indulged in by those with a constant supply of hot, running water. Unless Stew was given plenty of notice of a resident's intention to leave her nice warm flat, walk down the draughty verandah and risk catching pneumonia in the freezing cold bathroom, the chances were that nothing would happen when she turned the hot tap on, or there would be a tremendous banging in the pipes, sending shock waves shuddering through the building, followed by a rush of cold, rusty water, then nothing. The hot water system entirely depended for its success on Stew's conscientious stoking of the boiler. He often forgot to light it in the excitement of his latest journey into outer space.

But if Stew wasn't much good as a stoker he was a first-class furniture remover. He had learned the hard way from Mrs Peters. Twice she had stood, arms akimbo, directing operations while he and the old gardener moved her household effects from one flat to another. Neither of them had allowed an angry word to escape from his lips nor looked more than mildly frustrated when the three-piece cottage suite which they had pushed with much heavy breathing from one side of the room to the other had to be pushed back again. Stew had kept commendably cool while he was telling her that the dresser was a fixture and couldn't be moved from the living room into the kitchen. He maintained a dignified silence when she threatened to report him to the committee for placing a chair exactly where she had asked him, and he politely accepted the shilling she gave him as a reward for shifting the furniture and pandering to her every whim. The old gardener refused his shilling and when I reminded Stew that he wasn't supposed to take tips from residents he said he was only getting his own back. The shilling had fallen from his pocket when he was up-ending the sofa and he had seen Mrs Peters put her foot on it and pick it up when she thought he wasn't looking. In which case, he said, he had more right to it than she had. I apologized for almost accusing him of taking advantage of a poor old lady.

Moving Mrs Hunt didn't present nearly as many problems. She hardly flinched when the gardener dropped his end of the horsehair sofa that was being manipulated through the narrow doorway, and she didn't say a word when Stew dropped his end after they had scraped it onto the landing. She sat hunched on a three-legged stool, surrounded by carrier bags full of pots and pans, dishes and cutlery, and several bits of bric-a-brac. Two ashtrays piled up with stubs showed that she was quite content to wait until she and her carrier bags could join the rest of her belongings in her new little home on the lower floor. It was only when Stew dropped a chamber pot and the handle flew off that she started to take some interest in what was going on around her. She gave him a reproachful look and muttered a few naughty words.

'Not to worry,' he said cheerfully. It must have been cracked or the 'andle wouldn't have dropped off so easy. You want to think yourself lucky the whole thing didn't fall to pieces, the age it is.'

But Mrs Hunt didn't think herself lucky. She was greatly aggrieved at the mishandling of one of her most treasured possessions. Though she never had cause to use it, being still able to get to the lavatory in the night, it was a convenience she had no intention of being without. She said so to me, using more rude words.

'Don't worry,' I said soothingly, making allowances for the language. I knew that moving house could be a very stressful thing. 'I don't suppose he did it on purpose and as soon as you're settled in I'll go and buy you another out of petty cash.' I hoped the charitable body wouldn't grudge a shilling or two spent on keeping a resident happy. I had no idea then that the price of chamber pots had hit the ceiling.

Not far from the Lodge there was a shop which specialized in things that were no longer used for their original purpose and had become collector's items. Stone hot-water bottles stamped with the names of manufacturers long gone out of business kept company with candle snuffers, ear trumpets, warming pans and bashed-in copper kettles. Amongst these relics of the past were china chamber pots, patterned and plain. When I asked the man who owned the shop to wrap up a plain one and name his price, the price he named was more than a year's allowance for petty cash.

'But why are they so expensive?' I asked.

'It's the Yanks,' he said, putting the pot back on the shelf and folding the newspaper he had been about to wrap it in. 'There's a lot of them round here with the base being handy. They snap 'em up as fast as I can buy them in.' The Americans seemingly bought the pots to prove to the folks back home that England was as quaint as it had always been, and flush toilets hadn't yet crossed the Atlantic.

Mrs Hunt was so displeased with the bright blue plastic pot I bought from Woolworth's that Stew took her old one and glued the handle back on. He did such a good job that only the sharpest eye could detect the join.

Much later, when Mrs Hunt was no longer with us, the man who made a fortune out of selling obsolete items came to the flat and offered her family a very small sum for her stone water bottle, her warming pan, the bashed-in copper kettle, the candle snuffers, and the china chamber pot. When eventually they appeared in his window at greatly inflated prices Stew was as proud as a peacock at the thought that something he had almost invisibly mended was being offered as a genuine antique. He laid aside his science fiction and started gluing handles back on the old jugs and teapots he found in dustbins around the Lodge. He hoped that someday he would make a fortune out of them but as far as I know he never did.

It was after we had finished moving old Mrs Hunt downstairs that I discovered the nature of the affliction that had dogged Mrs Carter from her girlhood, and according to Annie had sent her husband to an early grave. When the last cup had been hung from a hook on the downstairs dresser and the last fluffy kitten calendar was securely pinned to the wall, I wandered wearily back up my garden path. There I noticed, not for the first time, that the riot of bindweed, the worn-out perennials and the exhausted biennials were in need of some attention. Never an enthusiastic gardener, I had to be in the mood for tackling such a major task. I hadn't been in the mood for ages, but I could ignore the riot no longer.

I was halfway to the compost heap, weighted down with weeds, when an emergency bell rang, followed in swift succession by others. Dropping the load I was carrying, and without stopping to wash my hands, I hurried across the forecourt.

A small group of women stood on the verandah, looking up at Mrs Carter's window. Through the window, which was an inch or two open, came the familiar squeals of anger and bursts of fury, reminding me that it was Tuesday and Annie had come to tea.

'You'd better get in there quick,' exclaimed Mrs Turgoose, who inevitably formed part of the group. 'They've been at it hammer and tongs since Annie got here but it's even worse than it usually is so we thought we'd better ring for you before they do each other a mischief.'

The other women nodded and stood aside for me to pass. The verandah was narrow and if there were more than three residents having a good gossip it was difficult to get past them without putting a foot in the gully. Stew spent a great deal of time clearing out the gully. Ladies who wouldn't have dreamed of dropping their litter where it could be seen by everybody had no scruples about blocking up the gully with their odds and ends. A lot could accumulate during a single gossip session.

I waited for a moment, hoping that the noise of battle would die down. When it didn't I wiped my hands down my skirt, pushed my hair in place and went upstairs.

Mrs Carter's door wasn't locked and when there was no reply to my knocking I walked in and approached the scene with caution.

The two sisters sat facing each other across the table. A snowy lace cloth, a few pieces of gleaming silver and some willow-pattern china lent an air of elegance to the battlefield. The sandwich plate was empty and a sizable wedge was missing from the cake. Both the sisters had little black caraway seeds stuck between their front teeth indicating that tea was over.

Annie's plump face was purple with anger. She had a butter knife in one hand and a cake fork in the other and was waving them both in a menacing way at her sister. Mrs Carter was armed with a teaspoon, her set face as white as the tablecloth. Neither of them knew I was there until I spoke.

'Ladies, ladies,' I cried, clapping my hands as if applauding their performance. 'You really must stop behaving like this. You can be heard across the fore-court and not only are you disturbing the other residents but I distinctly heard you using words which the charitable body wouldn't approve of.'

The two ladies stopped shouting and stared at me. Annie waggled her knife and fork within an inch of her sister's right ear. Mrs Carter instinctively dodged and put up her hands as if to ward off any blow that might be forthcoming. 'It's her you want to talk to,' spluttered Annie. 'She hasn't stopped getting at me since the moment I walked through the door. I've had about as much as I can take from her.' She lunged with the fork and Mrs Carter clutched at her head as though afraid she might lose it in the heat of the moment.

'I'm more than surprised at both of you,' I said sternly. 'It's disgraceful the way you behave on Tuesdays. What on earth are you quarrelling about this time?' Usually the quarrels were sparked off by some small barb aimed at a vulnerable spot.

'It's not me, it's her.' Mrs Carter stabbed her spoon into her sister's unbrassiered bosom. 'It's always the same when she comes for tea. She's never happy unless she's casting aspersions.' She paused for breath and patted the auburn topknot, poking in a few loose pins. Annie took advantage of the pause to pour out her version of the events that had led to my rushing post-haste from the compost heap.

'If there are any aspersions being cast round here it's her that's casting them as she always does.' She lowered her voice after I gave her a warning look. 'The other week it was the hat that I'd bought from Harrods, then it was my latest fur coat, and now it's my hair she's on about. She keeps insulting me by saying I have it dyed.'

I glanced at Annie's hair. The thin white line which ran along the centre parting stood out in sharp contrast to the inky blackness of the rest. It left no room for doubt that if the white line wasn't obliterated before Annie's next visit it would widen and show up even more sharply.

'I've always been proud of my hair,' Annie said. 'I used to be able to sit on it when I was a girl and it was as black as a raven's wing.'

'Well, it isn't black now,' snapped her sister. 'And as far as I can remember it never was. It was dead straight and a bit on the mousy side. You know as well as I do that it would be as white as the driven snow if you didn't have it done so regular. You must spend as much at the hairdresser's every week as I spend on food.'

Annie's face turned an even deeper purple. She jabbed with the butter knife again, Mrs Carter put her hands to her head and I spread out my arms in a gesture of peace.

'It's not a bit of use you carrying on like that,' said Mrs Carter, half rising from her chair. 'We both know that you've been having it done for years, ever since that coalman of yours started carrying on with the girl who used to work in his office. And being younger than you he'd have been off like a shot if he'd seen you as you really were. It was a blessing he went before he was any the wiser.' At this point I felt things had gone far enough. I braced myself to bring an end to hostilities.

'Well, I think you've both got lovely hair,' I cooed. 'I only wish mine was auburn or inky black instead of being pepper and salt like it is.'

The ruse worked. Both sisters looked pityingly at my uninteresting hair. Mrs Carter made another pot of tea and invited me to have a cup with them – and a slice of cake – after which I left them, at least quiet if not the best of friends.

I was lost in thought as I walked between the bindweed, the perennials and the other spent blooms. Though they were still running riot the afternoon hadn't been wasted. Not only had I brought peace, if only temporarily where there had once been strife, but I had learned the truth about Mrs Carter's affliction. I was amazed that it had taken so long.

When the battle of the cake fork, butter knife and teaspoon was at its height I had observed that whenever Annie lunged forward, threatening to strike, Mrs Carter shrank back as if to ward off the blow. It was during a particularly savage bit of infighting that the bright auburn cottage-loaf structure had slipped slightly to one side, revealing a hint of the baldness which was hidden from mocking eyes by the towering hairpiece. I should have known. The auburn had never sat easily amongst the faded ginger strands.

From then on whenever I was needed to settle a dispute between the two sisters I hurried across the forecourt dreading that Annie would do her worst and lay bare her sister's secret. But she never did. No matter how often her sister taunted her about the raven black hair that was as white as the driven snow at the roots she never retaliated by reminding Mrs Carter that she had no hair at all on top. I admired her for this. It couldn't have been easy for a woman of her temperament to bite back the words, and I wasn't surprised that the effort sometimes choked her and made her turn purple. There were times when I feared she was about to have a stroke.

But it was Mrs Carter who had the stroke. Her first was a mild one and she was able to ring her bell for me. It happened early in the morning. She was in bed when I got there, looking anxious and complaining of weakness in both her legs. She was wearing a lacy mob cap and out of the corner of my eye I saw the auburn hairpiece sitting on the bamboo table beside her bed. I pretended not to have seen it.

I had rung for the doctor when she pointed to the hairpiece. 'I want you to fix it for me before he gets here,' she said, removing the mob cap. I combed the faded strands of her own hair and pinned the more colourful pile on top, then I held a mirror in front of her to let her see if I had done it well enough for her. She gave me a twisted smile of approval.

'It looks nice,' I said. 'It would be hard to tell that it wasn't your own.' She gave me another little smile.

'There's not many that knows,' she said, in a slightly slurred voice. 'It's not something you go round boasting about like Annie does about her fur coats and her fine house on the common.' She was quiet for a moment and I gave her a lift up on the pillows and a sip of the tea I'd made.

'Have you been wearing it for long?' I asked her, already knowing the answer but wanting to take her mind off Annie's boastfulness and her own increasing loss of strength. I hadn't telephoned Annie. There would be time for that after the doctor had been. I hoped Mrs Carter was in no immediate danger.

'I've worn it since I was in my teens,' she said. 'I had a lovely head of auburn hair. It was a lot nicer than Annie's, which was always inclined to be greasy. And mine wasn't straight like hers. I can remember her sitting for hours under one of those perming machines when they first came into fashion, laughable it was to see her afterwards. Frizzed all over and scarcely able to get a brush or a comb through it. And as I've often told her, it would be as white as the driven snow by now if she didn't have it done. There's nothing I hate worse than to see a woman trying to look younger than she is.'

Mrs Carter gave a small sigh and I wondered if she had tired herself out with all the talking, but after I'd given her another sip of tea she started again. I let her go on. It seemed to be what she wanted.

'I started to lose mine after the young man I was engaged to was killed in the war – the first war, of course. We were going to be married on his next leave but it wasn't to be. Mother smothered me with everything when it started falling out but nothing made any difference. In the end she sent off to one of those places where they made wigs. I can't remember how much it cost her but it must have been a lot. It's real hair, which makes it look natural. I wouldn't be seen dead in one of those artificial things that Annie wears when she's going somewhere posh and hasn't had time to have her roots touched up. You can tell from a mile away that they're false.' She stopped talking and lay back on the pillows with her eyes shut.

Seeing the hairpiece at such close quarters I wondered again that I hadn't realized that it was Mrs Carter's affliction. But her flatlet was rather dark, she always wore one of her striped caps when she went out shopping, or her best hat for going to church and on the rare occasions when she visited Annie. I had accepted the bright auburn as a quirk of nature.

Mrs Carter opened her eyes again. 'I suppose I shouldn't talk about Annie the way I do,' she said, with a different note in her voice. 'She's been good to me in a lot of ways. She's often given me her cast offs – not that they were any good to me, her being the size she is. And she used to take me to the seaside for a day's outing once a year – but we got on each other's nerves, what with her throwing money away in the amusement arcades and not wearing stockings. We did nothing but fight so we stopped going. We've got on each other's nerves for as long as I can remember, though I have to say this much for her – she's never once cast up about me being bald on top, which goes to show there's good in the worst of us if you dig deep enough to find it.' Just then the doctor arrived to put an end to the short list of Annie's good points.

The first stroke didn't keep Mrs Carter in hospital for very long but the second one did. It kept her there for what remained of her life. The nurses on her ward were understanding about the hairpiece and made sure that it was firmly in place before the doctors and the matron did their round. But soon none of it mattered to Mrs Carter. She lay in a cot bed with rails up around it, not even recognizing Annie, who visited her every day, fed her with hothouse grapes, and wrapped bed jackets edged with swansdown round her poor thin shoulders. Neither did she notice that the white streak along Annie's centre parting got wider and wider until there was more of it than there was of the glossy black.

Annie never had her roots touched up again, and by the time her sister died her hair was as white as the driven snow.

Neither of the two more serious illnesses that Mrs Turgoose had while I was matron of the Lodge was serious enough to put her out of action for longer than a few weeks at a time, but she stretched them out, glad of the chance to be the centre of attraction while she could. Unlike her old enemy, Mrs Marsh, who had obstinately refused to go into hospital even when she knew she was dying, Mrs Turgoose went off as happily as was possible under the circumstances, exchanging a few double-meaning words with the ambulance men who came to fetch her.

As well as being willing to go into hospital she pulled strings that got her into convalescent homes. It was these periods of convalescence that made her illnesses so interesting.

After her first bout of pneumonia she spent two weeks in a place of recovery where she was the only patient who dropped her aitches and took her teeth out before she tackled her meals. Taking her teeth out and laying them on the table hadn't endeared her with the rest of the patients, most of whom were upper middle class. But she learned from the experience and when she returned to the Lodge she was not only a new woman healthwise but she had picked up a few refinements.

Though never going as far as wearing her teeth while she was eating, she attached heavy aitches to words that didn't need them and stuck out her little finger almost to breaking point when she drank a cup of tea. She cancelled her regular papers and ordered the less popular sort and she called me 'My deah' in a way that infuriated me. She eventually went back to being her normal, less than refined self, but not until she had alienated at least one resident with her delusions of grandeur.

Gladys Smythe, who had been her best friend for years, was deeply offended when Mrs Turgoose hinted that if she squirted stuff under her arms like the ladies did in the convalescent home it might stop her from smelling. Gladys buried her nose in her armpits and retorted angrily that if anybody needed stuff to stop them from smelling it was Mrs Turgoose. I was called in when deadlock was reached after they both ran out of insults. But I noticed afterwards, when I got close enough to Gladys's armpits to be able to smell them, that they had been given a rather large squirt of deodorant. I wasn't sure which I preferred, the earthy smell of sweat or the sickly sweet odour of whatever it was she was using.

Mrs Turgoose tried next to bring a touch of convalescent home class to old Mrs Hunt, but again she created ill feeling. A lady in the home had done all her chain smoking through an elegant jewelled holder. If Mrs Hunt were to do the same, said Mrs Turgoose, her fingers and the front of her hair wouldn't get so badly stained with nicotine. Mrs Hunt tossed her head and said that if Mrs Turgoose minded her own business instead of sticking her nose in other people's the Lodge would be a happier place. None the less, she wrote a letter to one of her daughters, asking her to bring a cigarette holder when she next came to visit, but after one or two puffs through the pink plastic holder she threw it away and went back to getting her hair and fingers stained, and smoking her cigarettes until the cork tips stuck to her teeth.

Mrs Turgoose tried to make other changes round the Lodge after she came back from the rest home for invalid gentlewomen. Until she went there she had thought rather poorly of people who involved themselves too much with things which had to do with religion. She had often told me that in her opinion religion could do as much harm as good. Take missionaries, for instance, she said, they went to foreign parts preaching about sin to folks who hadn't heard of it before, and if that wasn't putting wrong ideas into people's heads she for one didn't know what was. But a saintly lady at the rest home had pointed out bits in the Bible that had made her see things in a different light. She had particularly liked the story of Adam and Eve making aprons out of fig leaves. She'd never heard that bit before and it had opened up a whole new literary world.

She came back determined to convert Gladys Smythe by making her read a chapter every day. But Gladys was a very slow reader and after a couple of verses she gave up, saying that she couldn't make head or tail of all the begetting that went on in Genesis. Mrs Turgoose struggled until she got to Methuselah, then she gave up as well. But she was never as hard on missionaries after that.

The next convalescent home that Mrs Turgoose went to, after a second bout of pneumonia that came no nearer killing her than the first one had, was less of an upper-crust establishment. It was milling with ladies who dropped their aitches and took their teeth out to eat their meals. She looked round in disgust the first time I went to visit her. 'Common lot they are in here,' she said, crooking her little finger at an alarming angle while she drank her tea. I noticed that her mouth was uncomfortably full of artificial teeth. There was a Gideon's Bible lying open on her locker. I could only assume that she was demonstrating to the other patients that she was a notch or two above them on the social scale.

She was her old self when I went to see her again. Her bottom teeth were out and the Bible was back in the locker. She had formed a close friendship with Else who was in the bed next to her and shared her liking for a good joke with plenty of nudges and leering winks. They took it in turn to buy a daily paper and Mrs Turgoose shared with Else the things I bought for her. 'Smashing lot they are in here,' she said, beaming. 'Not like them in that other place who was frightened to smile in case they cracked their faces.' She dug Else in the ribs and they both collapsed with laughter.

At the end of their stay in the convalescent home Else and Mrs Turgoose had sworn to remain friends forever. They never saw each other again but Mrs Turgoose often told me the rude stories that Else had told her. They weren't very funny but they made a change from those she'd been telling me since I went to the Lodge.

As the years passed Mrs Turgoose lost some of the stamina which she had been proud to inherit from her very late father. Instead of going to the Darby and Joan club every afternoon in order to keep abreast with the current scandals, she sat at home most days and relied on others to bring her the news. When there was nothing for them to report she sat by her fire concocting her own little scandals or stood by her window waiting for me to go by.

'That girl's in the family way unless I'm very much mistaken,' she said when we were both standing at her window watching Mrs Peters's granddaughter walk past, miniskirted and pretty.

'You'd better not let Mrs Peters hear you say that,' I warned her, knowing that nothing was further from the truth. Mrs Peters was devoted to her grand-daughter, who belonged to the Guides and spent her spare time running errands for her grandmother and for others round the Lodge, and in the town.

Mrs Turgoose paid no heed to my warning and soon the verandah echoed with the sound of Mrs Peters defending the family honour. When I reminded Mrs Turgoose that I had told her what would happen she was unrepentant.

'Well, all I can say is that if she isn't expecting now she soon will be, wearing skirts that barely cover her bottom: leading men on. It's the same with all of them nowadays. You mark my word, if they don't get babies they'll get kidney trouble with nothing to keep the draught out when the wind blows.'

Reading the papers around about that time I saw statistics which seemed to prove that she had a point. Hospitals were reporting a rush of young women, admitted with things that could have been the result of the wind – or something – getting up their skirts. But Mrs Peters's granddaughter wasn't one of them. She suffered no ill effects and continued to wear miniskirts until they went out of fashion.

If the rumours that reached her ears were lacking in spice Mrs Turgoose added a little herself to improve the flavour. When she heard via the grapevine that old Mrs Hunt's youngest son's boy had been sent to New Zealand by the firm he worked for, she didn't believe a word of it and wasn't afraid to say so.

'If you believe that you'll believe anything,' she sneered on hearing the news. 'And if that's what they want the old lady to think then good luck to them. But if I know anything he didn't need no passport to get to where he's gone. It'll be Dartmoor, I shouldn't wonder, slouching about the way he did in them leather jackets of his.' Even when old Mrs Hunt showed her a postcard with masses of cloud where the top of Mount Cook should have been, Mrs Turgoose still argued. 'You can't go by cards,' she said. 'Just because it's got a New Zealand stamp on it doesn't say it had to come from there. I had a card the other day that had been posted in London and I know for a fact that my sister-in-law's daughter who sent it has never been there in her life. They just get somebody to post it for them to mislead people.' She and Mrs Hunt weren't on speaking terms for the next few days.

In spite of becoming rather less active Mrs Turgoose managed to be the first to tell me who, it was rumoured, would be coming to live in the flat which Mrs Hunt had vacated. 'I hear there's a man coming to live upstairs,' she said one day while she was sitting at her sink giving a bunch of sweet peas their weekly wash.

I said that I very much doubted it. What I meant was that I fervently hoped not. I had enough troubles without a man coming in and causing more. And after almost a century of sheltering elderly ladies I could hardly see the Lodge as a unisex establishment, though there was apparently nothing in the rules that said it was strictly for women.

Miss May was aghast when she heard the rumour. Her waxen face lost whatever tinge of colour it had.

'But surely the charitable body would never allow a man to come in here,' she wailed. 'They must see that it would be most improper. I would never get a moment's rest if I thought there was a man prowling about upstairs.' Her flat was immediately below the empty one. 'And supposing he were to pass by my window when I was having a good wash down?'

I pointed out that men frequently passed by her window but as it was draped with enough impenetrable curtaining to ensure maximum privacy I thought she need have no fears about that. But Miss May still trembled. Her knowledge of men was minimal. The thought of a strange one living in such close proximity made her come over queer and stay queer for several days. While I was putting her to bed and getting her ready for the doctor to call she told me of a terrible experience she had once had. In faltering tones she described the time when she quite forgot to turn off her television set before she started preparing for bed. She was down to her petticoat before she looked at the screen and saw Macdonald Hobley's eyes resting on her while he was reading the nine o'clock news. The shock had driven her to taking two doses of brandy.

The rumour about the man coming in died down and others took its place.

'I really do know now who's coming in,' said Mrs Turgoose eagerly. I fanned my face. It was the middle of June and we were sitting in front of her fire having a nice hot cup of tea. The flames leapt up the chimney and the room was like a furnace. Outside it was particularly warm for the time of the year.

'Who is it then?' I asked.

Mrs Turgoose drew her shawl round her shoulders and pulled her chair up closer to the fire. She had felt the cold a lot since her last bout of pneumonia.

'Well, it's not a man like they said it was going to be. It beats me how these rumours get about. It's that woman who used to keep a shop in the High Street.' She waggled her finger in the direction she thought the High Street was.

'Which shop?' I asked. The High Street was narrow and choked with traffic. There were shops packed tightly on both sides.

'The one that isn't there now,' replied Mrs Turgoose. 'It was pulled down years ago to make room for the other shop that took its place. It was all before your time but there's plenty round here that remembers it.'

'What sort of a shop was it?' I asked, thinking of the small millinery and drapery stores that abounded in every high street until big business took over, making all the high streets look alike.

'Well, I don't mind telling you it wasn't the sort of shop you bought your groceries from,' retorted Mrs Turgoose, with more than a touch of sarcasm in her voice. 'Nor was it one like old Miss Peddle's. Her what's just retired.'

She didn't need to remind me of Miss Peddle who had just retired. Her little shop had survived longer than other similar shops, only closing down when its owner, as diminutive as her shop, became too frail to give her customers the service they'd come to expect. Part of the service was a long-winded talk delivered by the proprietress, spectacles pushed down her nose to be looked over rather than through. The talk took in most of what had appeared in the local paper, and much that hadn't for fear of libel action. Anybody going into the shop for a bundle of firewood or a bar of scrubbing soap had to wait as patiently as they could while Miss Peddle clambered over bags of coal and pyramids of galvanized buckets to get to the place where she thought she kept the soap. Usually, and to her amazement, it wasn't there at all, but was eventually discovered somewhere quite different, hidden amongst mousetraps, pot menders, wire toasting forks and cast-iron trivets. Even when the soap was found and wrapped in old copies of the local paper, it wasn't handed over the counter until Miss Peddle had finished telling the customer – by now desperate to get away – the sad tale of her brother's latest operation, and the one before that.

Buying a box of matches could take up most of the morning if somebody she knew had just had a baby or had passed away in the night. The street wasn't the same after Miss Peddle's shop closed down.

The next to go had been the little shop opposite. It was run by two genteel ladies who did a roaring trade with their home-made bread pudding and faggots. Courting couples on their way to the pictures bought fat slices of cold bread pudding and a couple of faggots to eat while they watched the film. There was many a troth plighted over a faggot in the Odeon.

'The shop which the woman who's coming in here kept didn't sell anything,' said Mrs Turgoose. 'All she had to do was sit there waiting for customers and take their money off them. I can see her now sitting with her legs up inside that shop.'

'But if she didn't sell anything, why did she sit waiting for customers?' I asked, wishing that Mrs Turgoose wouldn't take so long getting to the point. I knew better than to try to hurry her. She would have clammed up and refused to say another word.

'That shop must have been a little gold mine,' she went on. 'I've known the time when there were as many as a dozen men queuing at the door, waiting for her to open.'

I gripped the cup I was holding. However lenient

the charitable body may have been with the small weaknesses confessed to by the residents when they were filling in their application forms, I doubted if they would be as lenient with a woman who had once kept a shop that had men queuing by the dozen waiting for the doors to open.

'It was her legs that did for her in the end,' said Mrs Turgoose. 'They were covered in ulcers and you can't go on doing a job like that with ulcerated legs. Especially when the business started looking up.'

'Did she have anybody to help her?' I asked, with visions of a very tired lady coping alone with the queues.

'Only after they made it illegal to do it on the streets.' I gripped my cup again. 'The last I heard of her she'd sold out to one of the big betting combines and had bought a bungalow. They pulled down the premises and built the shop that's there now. She should never have kept the business going after her husband died. Running a betting shop is no job for a woman. Especially when she's got bad legs.'

I relaxed my grip on the cup, feeling rather ashamed of the thoughts I'd been having about the woman who had once run a perfectly innocent betting shop.

I needn't have worried anyway. The lady who came into the empty flat had never kept a betting shop, nor did she have bad legs. Mrs Turgoose had, as usual, got the wrong end of the stick. The new resident had once been a subpostmistress. She had arthritis in both knees.

Part Three

Part Three

Chapter Seven

IN ADDITION TO the many and varied duties which
kept me busily employed at the Lodge there was an
annual excursion that gave me a great deal of
pleasure. Every Christmas I played the part of Santa
Claus in a very small way, and listened to a fresh lot
of stories while I took liquid refreshment of one sort
or another with elderly people in the town, men as
well as women.

Some time during December a member of the
committee brought me a bundle of envelopes, each
containing a formal greetings card, without holly or
robins, and one or two crisp new pound notes. There
was one note if the charitable funds were low that year
and two if the funds were swollen. It was my duty to
walk round the town and deliver the envelopes to the
chosen few entitled to them. The conditions for being
eligible for one were the same as the conditions upon
which the flatlets were allocated; applicants were

judged on their record of soberness, providence and the current state of their bank balance. Those who thought they qualified filled in forms and sent them to an imposing block of offices in the town, then waited anxiously to hear if their application had been successful. If it had, their names were entered in the ledger that I took round with me when I delivered the envelopes. Those who failed to get into the ledger tried again the following year, unless something had happened to make them quite out of the running.

Like many women of my generation, and many older than me, I kept different clothes for different occasions. The black nylon fur hat on top of my wardrobe was only taken down when I went to a funeral. Sometimes it stayed there long enough to have gathered a film of dust, but if a virus or a particularly harsh winter had taken its toll of the residents, the black hat could be in use far too often for my comfort. Kept free from dust in tissue paper was a rather splendid feathered creation that I wore for weddings and for going to church on Easter Sunday. Wearing it on Easter Sunday was a nostalgic throwback to my childhood when the village church was a riot of splendid creations, worn in a keenly competitive spirit.

Lying around in odd corners of my official residence was an assortment of less glamorous headgear. There

144

were shapeless old pixie hoods and battered felt pill-boxes, unfashionable, but handy to pull on when I dashed out to collect a prescription or buy a fillet of plaice for myself or one of the residents. Among the pixie hoods and pillboxes there was a bright red woollen confection, a cross between a balaclava helmet and a Scottish tam-o'-shanter. This I kept exclusively for delivering the Christmas envelopes. Not only did it keep my ears warm on the chilly journey round the town, but it gave a touch of seasonal colour to the rather dreary ensemble that I wore throughout the winter.

Those whose names were in the ledger were mostly men and women who were the backbone of the town in their younger days, and before anybody knew what a precinct was, they had worked hard, saved hard, and were justifiably proud when along with their neighbours they owned the semi they lived in. The semi had cost them every penny of £200, which gave them a strong sense of satisfaction at having something to show for their years of labour. They talked to me about the time when they were young and had strolled on summer evenings through lanes and across the fields. The fields and lanes disappeared when the planners moved in and turned the familiar into something quite unrecognizable.

'I remember the day' was the opening for most of the chats I had with the recipients of the charitable envelopes. And I, having lived in the town since the start of the Second World War, shared in the nostalgia by recalling the steam trains which used to run regularly from the little station that went when the concrete buildings started taking shape. We spoke of the tiny Catholic church which had been a landmark since the time it was built in what was then a quiet street and which now, by some miracle wrought by the planners, was on the opposite side of a grand new road, its bell drowned by the noise of the traffic. This for me was a sign of the times we were living in. Change was everywhere, and without a brick being moved the Roman Catholic church had gone from one side of the road to the other, though not ecumenically so.

Not everybody threw open their doors and greeted me warmly when I called with the Christmas envelopes. At some of the houses a suspicious eye appeared at the window, bolts were drawn, guard chains loosened, and finally the door creaked open just wide enough for a hand to reach out and grab the envelope. Then the door was slammed shut again leaving me, pen poised and ledger open, waiting for a signature that I wasn't going to get. I needed the signature. It proved to the charitable body auditors that I hadn't embezzled the Christmas present money. Those I didn't get I forged. I scrawled so many signatures in a shaky, spidery hand that I lived in terror until the end of the financial year, in case the forgeries were detected and I would end up in Holloway. But if my sins ever found me out I was never confronted with them and soon I stopped worrying and did rows of wonderful signatures sitting by my fireside in the dark winter evenings.

Creaking front doors, rattling bolts and guard chains weren't always to be taken as an indication that I wasn't welcome. More often they meant that the door was stuck fast, not having being opened since the last time I called. Regular visitors used the back entrance, sang out 'Is there anybody at home?' and walked in. Or they established their identity and were admitted after the living room had been hastily tidied up. I and others not so privileged, even though we were welcome, had to stand on the front doorstep while draught excluding sausage dogs were kicked aside and bobbled curtains pushed along poles.

Some that I visited at Christmas were struggling to keep up appearances. They clung proudly to the tradition of not letting anybody know their business. Too often this meant that they let nobody know their needs. Some lived on pittances when they were entitled to more. But if I dared to say this there was an embarrassed silence followed by a firm denial that they were in want. I caught glimpses of the want while I was listening to all that had happened since the previous Christmas. Grandchildren had got married, a favourite cat had had to be put down, a son had died. Snaps were brought out of weddings and christenings, and of views of foreign parts where it was becoming fashionable to go on holiday – so long as there was a package tour going that way. Sometimes I shivered as I listened, and was glad of the red woolly hat and the matching scarf and gloves. If there was a fire in the front room grate (not being a regular visitor I was usually shown into the front room) it was seldom enough to warm more than the knees of those nearest to it.

Looking down at me in the chilly rooms were large portraits of bewhiskered men, hair parted in an exact line down the middle, standing in poses which must have taken the photographer a great deal of time to get right. There were pictures of brides in bustles, their groom with an arm thrown casually across a manly chest, looking suitably proud of the prize he had won. There were massive gilt-framed likenesses of small girls wearing buttoned boots and stiffly starched petticoats. Their little brothers also wore buttoned boots and stiffly starched petticoats, which probably caused problems at a later date.

On one wall of a house I went to at Christmas there hung an extra-large portrait of a beautiful young girl, wearing a cloudy white dress and a smile reminiscent of the Mona Lisa.

'Who is she?' I asked the apple-cheeked old lady who was pouring tea from a grubby brown teapot into two grubby cups. She hadn't bothered to keep up appearances, as was shown by her grubby apron.

'Who do you think it is? It's me, of course,' she said, cross with me for not guessing. 'I was a dancer in those days.' Before I had time to doubt her word she got up and with one graceful movement proved that she was telling the truth. In the light of the sixty-watt bulb her face became the face of the girl in the picture, but when she sat down again she was a little old lady with apple cheeks. Seeing this I had a moment of panic, wondering what I would look like at her age. I still had a long way to go and already my face was different from the one in the photograph I'd had taken when I first went to be a nurse, to show my mother how splendid I looked in uniform. Time can be unkind to faces unless the framework is right. Mine wasn't built to last.

Many of the names in the ledger were of people I hadn't met until they were included in the Christmas list. But I felt I already knew them from the things Mrs Turgoose had told me. As usual she was a mine of information. Simply by dropping a name, and betraying no confidences, I got the history of every branch and twig of the family tree, from the cradle to the grave. I was grateful for this. It saved me from making too many embarrassing mistakes. The trouble with people who were once the backbone of the town they live in is that they have so many family connections in the town it can be dangerous to talk to them about anybody. I once talked at great length about a butcher whom I suspected of grossly overcharging for his inferior meat, only to discover that the woman I was talking to was the butcher's first cousin twice removed. He overcharged me even more after that for his inferior meat.

I was particularly indebted to Mrs Turgoose for telling me all she knew about Miss Moon. If she hadn't I might have got myself into yet another embarrassing situation.

Miss Moon had been Mrs Turgoose's best friend since Gladys Smythe blotted her copybook by getting romantically involved with Mr Jones at the Labour Party jumble sale. Though Mr Jones had died before anything came of the romance, Mrs Smythe was never as friendly with Mrs Turgoose as she was before he started taking her to the pictures every Monday, and sitting beside her in the coach when they went on outings. Miss Moon had taken to sitting next to Mrs Turgoose in the coach, and helping her with the crossword when they were together at the Sunshine Club.

'She's not a bad old stick, taking her all round,' said Mrs Turgoose when she was giving me the lowdown on Daisy Moon. 'She got let down when she was a girl but I, for one, never condemned her for it. As I always said, she wasn't the first nor wouldn't be the last to make a mistake. I've never been one to throw stones.'

I was amazed at hearing that Mrs Turgoose hadn't condemned Miss Moon for making a mistake. She was the first to throw stones at the young who made mistakes. Things had been different in her day, she said. There was none of this larking about in the streets after nine o'clock at night, roaming in droves, seeing what mischief they could get up to. Granted, there were those like Daisy Moon who made a mistake, but that was altogether different from the way things were today, with nobody turning a hair when a girl had a baby before she was married. In her day, she said, people had showed a proper shame when such things happened. She had known women who were so shocked when their unmarried daughters got into trouble that they kept them indoors as soon as it started to show and only let them out for a walk after dark so the neighbours wouldn't see the mistake growing bigger under a roomy coat.

'But surely the neighbours would know when the baby was born,' I said. Mrs Turgoose shook her head.

'Not if they didn't want them to know,' she said. 'In that case the girl was whipped off to an aunt or a grandmother, or even an older sister, and the baby was brought up as theirs, or it was adopted from birth and nobody any the wiser.' She could name names, she said, of people not a million miles away from the Lodge who would be surprised if they knew who their real mother was; she could also name names (and would have done if I'd let her go on) of people who had no idea who their father was.

Miss Moon had been let down twice, as I discovered the first time I called on her. Both her mistakes, now middle-aged, lived with her, tenderly cherishing their little spinster mother. They were large men, not over-blessed with brains but filling the house with their presence. They bumped into each other and knocked against the furniture when they brought the tea which their mother ordered for the kind lady who had come with the charitable envelope. I never had time to drink the tea. I was too busy admiring the things that were laid on the table for me to examine. Both the men had a hobby. One did fretwork; the other stuffed little dead birds and small wild animals which he searched for diligently amongst all that was left of the hedgerows around the town. He also trapped moles and there were usually a few skins hanging on a line in the kitchen between a lot of shrunken socks and some greyish vests and underpants.

Neither of the brothers was an expert at his particular craft. The living room was crowded with peculiarly shaped pipe racks, fretted three-legged stools and wobbly flower pot stands. The spaces not filled with fretwork were used to display the other brother's unprofessional efforts. There were several birds that I couldn't put a name to, and something that had once been a barn owl roosted uncomfortably beside a flattish cat. The cat, I was told, had been the family pet for so long that nobody could bring himself to bury it when it finally expired. It was for this reason that the brother who didn't do fretwork had gone to the library and borrowed a book on taxidermy. But try as he might, he could never quite capture the beauty of a bird poised for flight, nor the correct stance of a stalking cat. The creatures he stuffed always looked as if they had been run over by a heavy vehicle, which indeed some of them had.

The house next door was also on my list. The lady who lived there didn't welcome callers. When I rang her bell she came to the front room window, pulled aside the curtain and took a long look at me before she drew back the bolts and let me in. Not a word was spoken as she shuffled in front of me into the kitchen. There, she opened the envelope, and took out the contents, looking very aggrieved if there was only one note, and not too happy if there were two. She then climbed on a chair and lifted a cash box from the top of a cupboard. This she unlocked and placed the money in it, adding it to all the other money she had accumulated through years of pinching and scraping. She neither signed the ledger nor uttered a word that might have been taken as thanks. I was glad to hear her drawing back the bolts. With all that money in the box she couldn't afford to take chances.

The year came when I wasn't allowed across the threshold. I knocked for a long time before she appeared at the window and stared at me. When she realized who I was and what I was there for she came to the door, but she didn't open it. Instead, she put her hand through the letter box and grabbed the envelope off me. The following year her name had been struck from the list.

Miss Moon told me that when she hadn't heard the

woman next door raking out her ashes as she did every morning, she had carefully instructed her taxidermist son on the correct way of dialling 999. He did exactly as he'd been told and the police came round within minutes. They had quite a job gaining access.

The social workers got a very bad press for neglecting their duties and not making sure that the old lady was looked after properly. But there was nothing they could have done, short of breaking and entering. She had never asked for help, nor would she have accepted any. No matter who came to her door she stared at them through the curtains, then shouted through the letter box, telling them to go away. There was nothing else they could do.

'Ah well, it takes all sorts,' said Mrs Turgoose. I knew. I met a wide variety when I did the Christmas round.

Katy was well known to me even without her name being in the ledger. She lived in a small house by the river. Crippled with arthritis she hopped around the town like a sparrow, stopping to greet her friends and never once mentioning the severe pain she undoubtedly suffered. Questions about her health were answered with a wry grin and a cheery: 'Mustn't grumble, there's a lot worse off than me.' The way she said it gave sincerity to the trite phrase.

On the days when the arthritis got the better of her and she had to stay at home, she sat at her window and watched the swans, bottoms up, diving for food, or paddling across the road with their family tagging on behind. Every year a mating pair built their nest along the road, not far from where Katy lived. When the cygnets were hatched the proud parents held up the traffic several times a day while they walked in stately procession from nest to river. Cub reporters on the local paper, looking for a heart-warming story to fill up half a column when news was scarce, took notebook and camera down to the river and waited for the swans to provide them with material. Once, there was a different story for them to report, a sick sad story. When a family of cygnets was wantonly destroyed by hooligans with time on their hands Katy gave the newspaper men a graphic but unprintable account of the murder most foul. She refused to have her picture in the paper, along with an expurgated version, saying that the way they put it didn't in the least express the way she felt.

After her name was removed from the ledger it seemed as if yet another landmark had gone from the town. Her little house was turned into a modern maisonette and the road became too busy for the swans to nest in peace. They moved up river to a more select area and the reporters had to look for something else to fill a space when news was scarce.

There were married couples as well on the list. They also were of infinite variety. Some spent the time I was with them bickering and nagging as they had done throughout their married life. But I could see that the bickering had lost its bite and the nagging its sting. 'Father' grumbled if his dinner was served up late – or a minute too soon – and 'Mother' scolded 'Father' for not wearing his cardigan when he went out to fetch a scuttle of coal. Both pretended to be deafer than they were and it all ended happily, with Father giving Mother a peck on the cheek and Mother forgiving him for being a stubborn old man.

One such couple I visited were nearing their century. He was tall, lean, and ruddy cheeked. She was small, neat, and very bossy with him sometimes. When I visited them at Christmas a bottle and three glasses were brought out of the sideboard. Over a thimbleful of sherry they told me of the children they had lost in the past, of great-great-grandchildren who were starting to make their appearance and of naughty things they remembered doing back in their courting days.

It was usually he who did the remembering. 'Don't you believe him, he's having you on,' Mother protested roundly when Father gleefully told me something that must have been true; why else should she have turned pink at the memory and pretended to be cross with him for daring to say such a terrible thing? The twinkle in his eye belied his years and deepened her colour. Though she pushed him away she looked quite girlish when he tried to put his hand on hers by way of apologizing for teasing her so. I watched and listened, envying them, and marvelling that the old chemistry still worked and romance hadn't altogether gone out of their lives.

I had a small romance of my own one year, but nothing came of it. I didn't turn pink when an aging hand fumbled for mine, and I didn't start getting together a bottom drawer at the first hint of a proposal of marriage. I gave the proposal a few minutes' thought between one Christmas and the next but by then it was too late anyway. The gentleman had married somebody else.

I had been taking a charitable envelope for quite a few years to a widower who lived close to the Lodge. He had often told me how good he was at cooking, cleaning, and sewing on his own buttons. I had remarked on his highly polished lino and the excellence of the cake which he had made himself from a recipe his good wife had always used until she passed on, leaving him to fend for himself. Since he appeared to be fending for himself quite admirably I was all the more surprised when he pushed his chair closer to mine after he had signed the ledger.

'I was wondering whether you'd care to drop in for a game of cribbage one evening,' he said, closing the ledger with a slam and pocketing my pen. I had never played cribbage and told him so but he said that you were never too old to learn and it would be his pleasure to teach me. There was many an old dog who had been taught new tricks, he said. It was just a matter of master and pupil hitting it off.

I waited until the days lengthened before I took him up on his offer. I had noticed at Christmas that he rather favoured heavily shaded lights. This I felt could be a drawback when I was trying to get to grips with cribbage.

He produced a pack of cards, a cribbage board and a box of spent matches and started to give me my first lesson. His chair was very close to mine.

I was in the process of adding up nine and six on my fingers to make sure that they came to fifteen (a golden number in the game of cribbage) when he put all his cards on the table instead of just the one he should have done. I stopped counting, but held on to my cards.

'I suppose you've never thought of marrying again,' he said, edging his chair even closer and reaching out a hand in the direction of mine. I swiftly removed my hand and shook my head in a decidedly negative fashion.

'Pity,' he said. 'I've been looking round for a nice respectable woman somewhere about your age. This place needs a woman. However good a man may be there's still things he can't do for himself.' He gave me a nudge which reminded me of Mrs Turgoose. 'And you could do worse, you know. I don't drink and I don't smoke and I've got a bit put by besides the old age pension.' He picked up his cards again. 'Anyway, give it a bit of thought and it's your deal.'

I gave only a fleeting thought to the prospect of having to polish the lino to his rather pernickety standard, baking cakes as delicious as those which his good wife used to bake, and spending long winter evenings counting up fifteen on my fingers. But before I got round to giving him my answer Mrs Turgoose told me that one of the old boys who went to the Darby and Joan club was getting spliced the following week. 'He's got one foot in the grave and so has she,' she said. After further derogatory remarks about the happy couple who were shortly to be married at the registry office she said something that caught my attention.

'He's been going round to her place a lot lately,' she said. 'She's told them that sits next to her at the club that he's been showing her how to play crib, but if you ask me he's been showing her a bit more than that.' She closed one eye and dug me in the ribs.

I didn't tell a soul about the evening I learned to play crib. It would almost certainly have got back to Mrs Turgoose and she would never have let me live it down.

Chapter Eight

IN SPITE OF the trouble everybody took to get old Mrs Hunt into her downstairs flat she never settled there. On the very day she moved she rang her bell twice, the first time to complain that the water tasted different down there from what it did upstairs and it was already giving her diarrhoea, the second time to tell me that because everything was the wrong way round in her new flat she kept going to the larder thinking it was the lavatory. Even having the freedom of the verandah wasn't nearly as much fun as she thought it would be. After a day or two of putting her head round the door and greeting everybody who walked past the novelty wore off and she sat huddled against the fire, no more adventurous than she was when she lived upstairs. Soon she was blaming me for ruining her life and forcing her to do something which she had never wanted to do.

'You should have minded your own business and let

me stay where I was,' she grumbled peevishly when I was giving her something for the diarrhoea. It had persisted even though I had done as Mrs Hunt asked, and filled up her kettle, several jugs, a teapot or two and an old plastic bucket with water from the upstairs flat. 'I'd lived in that little place for going on twenty years and it was as if I'd been born there. I shall never get used to being down here, stuck in a corner where I can't see anything. Up there I used to spend hours at the window watching folks coming and going. I might as well be dead as living here.' I tried not to think of the nights I'd lain awake wondering where I was going to put her after she insisted on being moved downstairs. I lay awake often worrying over things which turned out differently from the way I expected.

'I still think it's better for you to be down here,' I told her, handing her the cigarettes she'd asked me to go out and buy for her. 'And when the weather improves you'll be able to go and buy your own cigarettes, so long as you take care crossing the road.'

The road she would have to cross if she ventured out was very dangerous, with a constant stream of traffic that paid little heed to old ladies trying to get from one side to the other. I sent in a petition once, signed by the residents, asking whether some sort of device couldn't be placed near the entrance to the

Lodge that would halt the traffic long enough for the opposite pavement to be reached without lives being endangered. The reply was not encouraging. After sifting through the official language I gathered that since there had so far been no lives lost on the particular stretch of road to which my letter referred it was not thought necessary – or indeed advisable – for anything to be put there that would interrupt the flow of traffic. The writer went on to assure me that in the event of a fatality at some future date the situation would be reviewed by the appropriate department. For what could only have been a good reason the situation was never reviewed.

Mrs Hunt lit a cigarette, enveloping herself and me in a cloud of smoke. Already the cupboards, the ceiling and the curtains, sparklingly fresh when she first moved in, were starting to turn a delicate sepia. Soon they would be tobacco brown as those were that she had left behind.

'I don't feel like going anywhere these days,' she said wearily. 'I must be getting old.' She was already ninety-two. 'I haven't the go in me like I used to have.' She stubbed out her cigarette and lit another. She was stubbing out that one when I left her.

On her ninety-third birthday her daughter came to see me, looking very worried. 'I've been trying to tell

Mother that she'll have to leave here and come and live with one of us.' She sounded as if the telling hadn't been easy. 'We've been nagging her for years but it's been like talking to a brick wall. Well, now she'll have to listen. It's not fair on us, her being here at her age. What if she went suddenly and none of us was with her? People would say we'd been neglecting her all these years.'

I knew that Mrs Hunt's family had never neglected her. And I knew how much they had nagged her. She used to get very cross when she told me about it.

'To hear that lot talk anybody would think I wasn't capable of looking after myself,' she said, when her family went home after another session of nagging.

'They're only trying to do what's best for you,' I told her, knowing that I was wasting my breath.

'What's best for me is to be left to do as I like. It's all right for them to talk but I'm not used to that fancy stuff they eat and the way their kids carry on. And since that oldest son of mine gave up smoking he goes round with one of them air fresheners every time I have a fag.'

'What about your daughter?' I asked. Mrs Hunt pulled a long face.

'She's as bad as him,' she said. 'She's frightened to death in case I drop ash on her carpet. As far as I can make out it sets fire easy.'

'There's your youngest son,' I said. 'He's ever so fond of you and you'd be happy there.'

'That I wouldn't,' she said. 'I'd never last a minute with that lad of his playing his guitar till all hours of the night. It's enough to deafen anybody if they're not deaf already.' Her youngest son had been deaf and dumb since he had meningitis when he was a very small boy.

'But they've already told you that if you make up your mind to go and live with them you could have the room at the back where you wouldn't hear a thing.' She gave a derisive snort, forcing the smoke down her nose and making me have to pat her on the back to stop her from choking.

'I'd need a room at the bottom of the garden as well as a pair of ear plugs if I went to live with them.' She wiped her streaming eyes. 'I get enough of it when I go there on Sundays, without having to put up with it for the rest of my life. It wouldn't be so bad if it was only him, but he brings his mates in at night and they wind up that gramophone and have things like yeah yeah yeah blaring out all over the house. They say it's beetles but it sounds more like cats screeching to me.' I had to admit that even to my rather younger ears the Beatle sound had none of the dulcet notes for which Tauber was famous.

Mrs Hunt was still asserting that no power on earth would make her leave the Lodge, when one morning a higher power intervened and she quietly left the Lodge. One of her daughters was with her when it happened. When I hurried to answer the bell she was sitting holding her mother's hand.

'Ah well, I suppose it was for the best,' she said, putting the frail old hand together with the other. 'We all knew she'd never have settled with us, and she was happy here, even if she did complain about having to come downstairs. She spent some of the best years of her life in here, what with Dad drinking himself to death and leaving her with us lot; and one of the boys being deaf and dumb. She's never had it easy. It's nice to think she went quietly in the end.' She gave a little laugh. 'I didn't know she'd gone until I saw smoke coming up from the carpet where she'd dropped her cigarette. Typical of her, that was. We always said if she didn't go grumbling she'd go with a fag in her mouth.'

We emptied the ashtrays and did other things that had to be done, then the daughter went off to break the news to the rest of the family. I stood for a moment looking at Mrs Hunt and thinking that death didn't seem nearly so awful when it happened to an old lady while she was sitting in her chair, happily smoking a cigarette, as it had done when Mrs Smith's grandson died of leukaemia when he should have been sitting for his O levels. The relatives would accept it without asking me or anybody else why such things were allowed to happen. Mrs Smith asked the question often after her grandson died.

Not everybody at the Lodge asked why such a thing had happened or blamed the Almighty for letting it happen. Mrs Dean, who was always losing things and putting the blame on others, lost a daughter and blamed nobody but herself.

Mrs Dean had three sons as well as the daughter who died. She was a possessive mother and the sons took years to pluck up enough courage to tell her that they were going to marry the girls who had waited patiently for them to make up their minds. After the last one had gone the mother tightened her hold on her daughter, determined that at least one of her children should stay dutifully at home, and be a comfort to her until the day she died. With this always in mind she put her small foot down firmly whenever her daughter showed signs of forming an attachment with a presentable young man. The two women settled down to what looked like being an uneventful life together while Mrs Dean lived, followed by an even duller existence for the daughter when she was left alone.

They got on reasonably well with each other. There were the inevitable small differences: whose turn it was to get up first and make the morning tea, and who had made the hot chocolate the evening before; whether one should weed the garden while the other cooked the lunch, or if both should weed the garden and leave the lunch to cook itself. Occasionally a little bitterness crept into the conversation when the daughter remembered the nice young men who came to court her but who had abandoned the idea after it was brought home to them that there would always be a third party present at the courtship. Mrs Dean kindly volunteered to make up a threesome if they were going to the pictures, and insisted on joining them when they went for a day in the country. She smiled sweetly and brought out the canasta cards if the young men looked like staying after supper. The sons had fought to the bitter end against the canasta cards and had emerged from the conflict so weak that they never fought again. They were as putty in their wives' hands and did the washing up without ever having to be asked twice, wearing the plastic pinny with the slogan on which they got for Christmas. They were model husbands.

But nothing went according to Mrs Dean's plans. Fate had other things in store for her daughter. Miss

Dean flustered home one Sunday lost in a dream of romance after a burly middle-aged man had raised his hat to her when she was sitting feeding the ducks in the park. She went to the park most days while her mother had her afternoon nap, and took a slice or two of bread to throw to the ducks. The man had sat down on the other end of the bench and said how nice the weather was for the time of the year. From this small seed love blossomed for Mrs Dean's daughter.

It was almost a year before the burly man had inched his way up the bench in the park, until he was sitting close to Miss Dean, and almost another year before they tore down the barriers of shyness and talked of other things than the weather. But by then they both knew that they were made for one another. A friend of the family asked Miss Dean how she could have been so sure that the man in the park wasn't married, and she replied that anybody as nice as he so obviously was would have brought his wife with him instead of coming alone with bags of stale bread to give to the ducks. When the question gave her little nagging doubts she popped into the library on her way to the park and looked him up on the electoral roll. There were no women living at the address he had written down on a page torn from his diary, and no other men either. From which she rightly assumed that he was unattached and perfectly at liberty to court her, as he clearly intended doing.

Meanwhile Mrs Dean slumbered under her eider-down, totally oblivious of what was happening in the park down the road. She hardly bothered to listen when her daughter touched lightly on the man who talked about the weather and other things in his quiet way. She went on buttering the scones for tea as if Cupid wasn't threatening her future with his bow and arrow. But suddenly Miss Dean grew reckless. She threw caution to the wind and in one long gulp confessed to what she had been doing in the park for the past two years. She explained about the ducks, the stale bread and the park bench, and eventually got round to the man who had edged his way along it, inch by inch. She stood her ground when her mother collapsed into the nearest chair and asked brokenly what would become of her, her ungrateful sons gone off to live with other women and now her only daughter talking of deserting her. It was her future son-in-law who supplied the answer to that. He had already given the question his earnest consideration.

'How about putting in for a flatlet down at the Lodge?' he asked Mrs Dean while they were playing canasta one evening. Unlike the sons he never minded playing canasta, preferring it to turning out on a cold night to go to the pictures. His future mother-in-law used most of the playing time putting obstacles in the way of his marrying her daughter but he played on doggedly. He gave her time to stop swooning at the thought of living at the Lodge, then he listed the advantages. It would be better, he said, than living in a four-bedroomed house all by herself after her daughter got married – she swooned again but he carried on regardless – and infinitely better than moving in with any of her children and being a guest in their house, however welcome, rather than mistress of her own.

He spoke from the heart. He had never been married before and though he liked Mrs Dean he preferred not to share his wife with her if there was any alternative. He had listened when men were talking about their mothers-in-law and from the things they said had deduced that distance was required if there was to be any closeness between them.

Just to make sure, the man who was going to marry Miss Dean wrote himself to the charitable body asking for an application form for a flatlet. When it came he sat beside Mrs Dean and helped her to fill it in. He did it in such a kindly way that by the time they had come to the bit about her being sober and provident she had grown quite fond of him and was able to smile weakly at his little joke about her soberness.

When her signature had been appended on the bottom line she took a bottle of ruby wine from the sideboard where it had stood since the previous Christmas and poured out three glasses, thereby making it a sort of celebratory occasion.

It was while they were sipping the wine that Miss Dean's affianced told them that his granny had lived at the Lodge many years ago. He remembered his mother taking him to see her. He had liked going there. The old ladies had given him toffees which had often tasted of camphor balls, and those with budgerigars had allowed him to put his finger in the cage and stroke the downy little heads. But that was a long time ago, when old ladies were very old ladies and wore clothes which stamped them as being decidedly of a past generation. These days, he said, looking at Mrs Dean, there was nothing to tell mother and daughter apart. On the strength of this she gave him another glass of ruby wine.

He also recollected his granny telling his mother, though he shouldn't have been listening, that the matron who was there at the time was a proper old cow. Mrs Dean looked pained and he begged her pardon for using the expression. The pardon was granted and he went on to tell all he remembered of the things his granny had said. According to her the matron had marched round every morning, opening cupboard doors and looking under beds to make sure that none of the residents had a man hidden there. She was a stickler for rules, to put it politely, and the rules said that on no account must the residents harbour men, either in their cupboards or under their beds. She was as fanatical about that as she was about residents who took a drop too much and staggered along the verandah on Saturday nights singing at the tops of their voices.

'I suppose your granny's name didn't happen to be Sal?' I asked Miss Dean's intended, when he was telling me about the past while measuring up the flatlet her mother would be moving into. He thought hard for a moment, then said that he seemed to remember her name being Sarah and it was quite probable that her friends had called her Sal. Would she, I asked, by any chance be the same Sal who was sent from the Lodge in disgrace for singing on Saturday nights after she'd had a few? Again he thought hard. Yes, he said, now he came to think of it he remembered his mother telling the neighbours that his granny had left the Lodge in a hurry after the matron reported her to the charities for breaking the rule which said that residents should at all times be sober and orderly. Apparently his granny was never sober, at least not on

Saturday nights, and she ended her days up at the infirmary, where she had bottles of stout smuggled in on visiting days by her old drinking pals.

When he asked how I came to know so much about Sal since it had all been long before my time, I took him to see Mrs Turgoose. She had been his granny's best friend before they came to the Lodge, and right up to the time when Sal was slung out for disorderly conduct. He had a little chat with Mrs Turgoose and it all came back to him. He recalled how his mother had blamed Polly Turgoose for setting his granny's feet on the road to ruin. It had all begun on the day his granddad was buried.

His granddad, it seemed, hadn't been the best of husbands and the marriage had been a stormy one. After his funeral Mrs Turgoose took Sal and the other mourners for a port and lemon at the pub next to the cemetery. The party had got a bit out of hand and many of the mourners ended up in the Black Maria. His mother, he said, hadn't been able to hold her head up in church after that and had come within a hair's breadth of being expelled from the Mothers Union.

Mrs Turgoose got very upset when I mentioned the funeral and the Black Maria. Never in her life, she said, had she ever set foot in anything so disgraceful. She threatened to sue Sal's grandson for defamation of character, and me as well if I didn't knock the story on the head before it got all round the Lodge. It took two cups of tea to calm her down, and another two to make her confess that she was at the party on the day that Sal's husband was buried, and might even have been bundled into the Black Maria with the other mourners.

'But you don't drink,' I said. 'I thought you only had a glass or two of sherry at Christmas, a drop of gin when it was somebody's birthday and a slurp of sweet wine at the Masonic Christmas dinner, to wash the turkey down.' She fiddled with a vase of plastic gladdies that had lost their colour through being washed too often.

'Yes, well,' she said, sounding embarrassed. 'Sal deserved a bit of a treat after her old man went. He used to knock her about something shocking and it was a relief to all when he fell in the canal on his way home from the Swan one night. I was thick with Sal in those days and after we were both made widows we used to go regular for a bit of a singsong on Saturday night. Then we had a row and I stopped going with her so much.'

The turning point in the friendship came when Sal started an argument while she was entertaining a few friends in her kitchen. The argument brought not only the Black Maria but a fire engine and an ambulance as well to her door. Mrs Turgoose was laid up for a week with bandages and bits of sticking plaster everywhere. She came out of hospital vowing that never again would she be a prop for Sal to lean on when her knees buckled beneath her. This wasn't to say, said Mrs Turgoose, that they had stopped being friends but Sal had to find somebody else to go out with on Saturday nights. Mrs Turgoose hadn't seen the inside of a Black Maria from that day to this.

'She was her own worst enemy,' she said sadly of Sal. 'Even she should have had more sense than to come in the worse for wear when she knew that old cow of a matron was only waiting to have her chucked out. She could have been here still like me if she'd contented herself with a drop of gin now and again.'

The marriage between Miss Dean and the man she met in the park took place quietly. Mrs Dean moved into the Lodge and except for suddenly starting to lose things and blaming others for robbing her she seemed quite happy. She even forgave her daughters-in-law for marrying her sons, and when her daughter surprised everybody by having a baby when they all thought she was past it Mrs Dean doted on the tiny mite and lived in constant fear that it would be mysteriously mislaid, in the manner of Mrs Dean's belongings, and turn up in some unlikely place.

But the baby thrived and was a sturdy schoolboy when both his mother and his father were killed in a car crash.

'It's my fault,' said Mrs Dean when her sons came to tell her what had happened. 'I should have kept her at home with me instead of letting her get married.' It took a touch of the supernatural to change her mind. But that wasn't until much later.

Chapter Nine

IF BEING THE matron of the Lodge gave me little scope for performing deeds of heroism or practising the more advanced techniques of nursing, neither did I get much experience in dealing with crime. Until Miss Silver came to live with us I had only read about the things she did; I had never met anybody who actually did them.

Because it was Miss Macintosh who told me that Miss Silver had started doing some rather peculiar things when she went shopping in the town, I knew that it was no idle gossip I was listening to. She would never have mentioned the matter if she hadn't thought it was serious. Unlike Mrs Turgoose, she wasn't the sort of woman to turn an insignificant little happening into a Lodge-shaking event. Mrs Turgoose had elaborated on a small adventure I once had until I began to wish I had never mentioned it to her. It had concerned three young men who scaled a wall and confronted me on the forecourt as I was going back to bed at two in the morning, after giving Miss May a cup of something to stay her. But the young men were more afraid of me than I was of them. They looked at me, fearsome in dressing gown and pyjamas, and climbed back over the wall as fast as they could.

Mrs Turgoose had passed on the story after I told her about it. When it reached Mrs Peters it had grown so much in stature that Mrs Peters was convinced that she had barely escaped being murdered in her bed. 'I've been expecting something like this to happen,' she said darkly. 'Which is why I always keep these handy just in case.' In a corner by her bed were two brass pokers with enormous knobs. A single blow from one of the knobs would have shattered the thickest skull. 'Be prepared is my motto,' said Mrs Peters. 'I've never let anybody take advantage of me, nor never shall while there's breath left in my body.' She looked defiantly through her window and threw back her shoulders, as if to warn anybody waiting to take advantage of her that he waited in vain.

Miss May had been gratifyingly appreciative of the fight I'd put up to save her from death or worse. 'Dear brave matron,' she breathed, pressing grateful kisses into the palm of my hand. 'How can I ever thank you for saving my life?' I told her not to mention it,

assured her that it was all part of the job, and gave her
some brandy before the thought of what could have
happened made her come over queer. It took two stiff
doses to give her the strength to drink her Milo.

Miss Macintosh was Scottish. She was a quiet, reti-
cent lady, often accused by her neighbours of being
standoffish. Shortly after she came to live at the Lodge
a rumour spread that she had inherited a great deal of
money. The rumour was false but Miss Macintosh
never lived it down. Not only was she accused of
having money, but being Scottish she was accused of a
decided reluctance to part with it. If she was seen
wearing something new, those watching behind their
net curtains muttered things about people as rich as
she was taking up a flatlet that was intended only for
those in reduced circumstances. If she went out
wearing the coat she had worn for years, harsh things
were said about her meanness. But none of this troubled Miss Macintosh. She had long since forgotten
that the distant cousin who left her wealth to a donkey
sanctuary was supposed by some of the residents to
have left it to her.

She had a soft brogue that could sharpen considerably when she was telling the milkman that he had
charged her for a pint she hadn't had. But when she
was sitting beside a bed saying comforting things to a

sick old lady, the brogue flowed as gently as a Highland stream.

Miss May was devoted to Miss Macintosh. She was devoted to anybody who preferred to listen rather than talk and Miss Macintosh was a most patient listener. She never minded how often Miss May told her the tragic story of her younger days, when her ailing father had taken to his bed leaving four sickly daughters and a worn-out wife to cope without him. He had died when Miss May was barely in her teens. Her mother followed soon after.

Only one of her sisters ever got as far as the altar and the man she married entered into the state of matrimony with his eyes wide open. He had known from the start that there would be four little women for him to cherish (if not to have and to hold) instead of just the one he had promised to endow with all his worldly goods. Being chronically short of worldly goods, he moved in with his bride and her sisters and shared the work in the hand laundry bequeathed to them by their mother. Not only did he help with the washing, mangling and ironing, but he attached a large wicker basket to the front of his bike and pedalled furiously though the town collecting and delivering the linen of rich citizens who could afford to pay a penny to have a shirt or a sheet hand laundered.

Being a kind-hearted man he saw to it that all four women got a fair share of his attentions. He would never have dreamed of leaving one of them out if he was planning a little excursion to the shops, and he bought them little treats while he was delivering the laundry.

As a husband he was peerless. When his brand-new bride complained of a headache brought on by the excitement of getting married, he obligingly suggested cancelling the honeymoon. Instead of taking her to the seaside for a long weekend he took her home and looked on anxiously while her three sisters took it in turns to lay vinegar cloths on her brow and give her sips of brandy to steady her nerves. When they shyly pointed out to the brand-new groom that in the state she was in it would be foolhardy for her to have the upheaval of moving from her old room into the double room above the parlour, he quite understood. With tender consideration for her feelings he agreed to sleep there alone until such time as she felt able to creep in beside him.

It was a long time before she felt able. She had never in her life slept anywhere but with Miss May. The thought of leaving her dearest sister with nobody to turn to when she came over queer in the night so saddened her that she would willingly have put the honeymoon off for ever. Even when she at last steeled herself to kiss her sisters goodnight and take her rightful place beside her husband, one of her sisters, and maybe all three, would steal in to make sure she had everything she needed. One would find an extra shawl or another blanket, the other a pair of bedsocks to ward off chilblains, and the third would insist on making the happy couple another cup of cocoa. When these needs had been supplied they would sit on the bed and have long sisterly chats until they were all too sleepy to keep their eyes open a moment longer. If the sister's husband had any thoughts on this he kept them to himself. He was too fond of them all to risk hurting their feelings.

Miss May had once told me that if a visitor descended upon them and needed a bed for the night – or longer – it was always she who gave up her room and slid in beside her married sister, on the far side of the bed from her brother-in-law. When I asked her if he hadn't minded having three in a bed she hesitated before she answered. He hadn't exactly minded, she said, but he always insisted that she left her hot-water bottles behind. There had been one occasion, she said, when he got up in the night for something or other and had climbed back on Miss May's side instead of her sister's. He had apologized profusely for making such a silly mistake and as far as she could remember it hadn't happened again.

Miss Macintosh heard so many sad stories about the four little washerwomen that the gentle Scottish lady often stumbled back to her flat with tears in her eyes. One had been almost blinded by some terrible affliction, another had a chest complaint that wasn't helped by the long hours she spent in the steam laundry. The one who got married had faded away as her father had done, and only Miss May was left. She remained with her brother-in-law until he also died, then she sold the laundry and came to live at the Lodge. According to Mrs Turgoose, even after the laundry was modernized the women who worked in it said that when the machines had stopped and all was quiet, those brave enough to stay behind until darkness fell heard the creak of a mangle and the swish of an iron, and sometimes a distant sound of voices as if Miss May and her sisters still chattered over the washboards.

Knowing Mrs Turgoose's gift for invention I took the story of the haunted laundry with a pinch of salt.

I had gone up to thank Miss Macintosh for being so kind to Miss May when she started to tell me what she had seen Miss Silver doing in the town.

'I saw Miss Silver in the town this morning when I

was doing my shopping,' she said, trying to sound casual.

'She walks into the town most mornings,' I said, wondering why such an apparently useless piece of information should have been passed on to me. Miss Macintosh nodded thoughtfully.

'I know she does,' she said. 'I just thought you ought to know that she's started doing some very peculiar things.'

'What sort of things?' I asked.

'I hate to say it, but she's started taking things off the shelves and walking out without paying for them.'

I sat down quickly on the nearest chair, feeling dazed. I was already seeing terrible times ahead if others had noticed Miss Silver helping herself in the serve-yourself shops. There would be headlines in the paper and policemen milling round the Lodge, not to mention the things the committee would say when I was hauled over the coals for neglecting my duties in not seeing that Miss Silver did her shopping in an orderly fashion.

'Are you sure about this?' I asked Miss Macintosh, hoping against hope that she had made a mistake. She was well over seventy and it wasn't unreasonable to think her eyes might have played her a trick.

'Quite sure,' she said firmly. 'I've followed her round

the supermarket all this week and she's been piling things into her shopping bag as if she didn't care a hoot whether anybody saw her or not. Then she's walked straight past the checkout and through the door.'

'And what happened to the things she took?' I asked.

'I didn't know what to do without making a fuss. So I've been going quietly up to her and offering to carry her bag. She's never seemed to notice that I took the bag back into the shop and brought it out empty. I had to be careful when I was replacing the goods but there aren't many customers about early in the morning and the assistants are either standing about in corners gossiping, or sticking fresh price labels on things as they do every day. But I think something will have to be done about Miss Silver before she gets into trouble.'

I thanked Miss Macintosh for the tactful way she had dealt with a difficult situation and went home to think how I should deal with it. I had already had reports about Miss Silver's strange behaviour, but this was the first I'd heard of her shoplifting. I tossed and turned that night looking for a solution to a new and rather frightening problem.

Miss Silver had come to the Lodge after her bachelor brother died and left the family house to his favourite nephew who had only just got married and wasn't happy at the thought of getting an aunt thrown in with the house. He had nothing against her, he said, but he didn't think it would work. The way he saw it, and no disrespect to the old lady, every young couple should be given the chance to get used to being married without having a third party interfering all the time. Miss Silver said she quite agreed and would be perfectly happy going to live at the Lodge.

Until she retired she was a subpostmistress in a rather seedy part of the town. She had been happy in her work. Like Miss Peddle in her little shop, Miss Silver never sold a stamp without entering into a long and rambling discussion on the events of the week. She sat behind the grille handing out pension money, family allowances and plenty of good advice. Then one day a man burst into the post office, pointed a gun at her and told her to hand over the takings – or else. She didn't wait to find out what 'else' meant. She threw a scalding hot cup of tea at the man and he fled before she had time to hurl the saucer. He was still having treatment for his burns when they caught him.

She was pensioned off and given a framed letter from the Postmaster General saying how grateful he was to her for showing such courage and having the presence of mind to throw the tea. She was never the same again, but she had seemed perfectly normal when she came to live at the Lodge, and had never mentioned the man with the gun.

Miss Cromwell had been the first to complain about the way Miss Silver was behaving. She had pounded up my garden path, her face dark with anger. She was wearing her round black hat, her black plastic raincoat, her grey stockings and a pair of sturdy black shoes. Even I had to admit that she looked a bit like a matron.

'I just caught that woman who lives above me trying to get into my flat,' she stormed, the black hat almost falling off under the pressure of her emotions.

I understood her anger. Nobody was allowed in Miss Cromwell's flat, let alone a resident making an unauthorized entry. When I did a round the door was opened just wide enough for me to see a notice that was propped between two china dogs on her dresser. The notice said: 'Please keep out and don't come in.' Neither I nor anybody else had been known to flout the injunction.

'I expect it was all a mistake and Miss Silver thought she was getting into her own flat,' I said, trying to calm Miss Cromwell before she started foaming at the mouth.

'How could she have thought that when she's

upstairs and I'm downstairs?' asked Miss Cromwell, with reason on her side. I said I didn't know but I'd try to find out. She went up the path and out of the gate at her usual cracking pace.

Miss Silver stoutly denied doing anything so outrageous as trying to get into somebody else's flat. 'I wouldn't stoop so low,' she said, very indignantly. 'I'm not one of those people who go around having cups of tea with people then threatening them with guns.' I gave her a sharp look but she trotted off into the kitchen and came back with a packet of biscuits which she insisted on giving me to prove that she bore me no malice for thinking ill of her. When I tried to refuse them she assured me that there were plenty more where they came from. I took the bourbons home and ate them one by one, unaware that I was committing an offence.

A week or two went by before Miss Silver again tried to gain entrance into somebody else's flat. Miss Macintosh rang her bell for me and I found the two ladies sitting by the fire enjoying a cup of tea, some ginger biscuits and a cosy chat. Miss Macintosh closed one eye in a conspiratorial wink.

'Miss Silver thought she would come to the post office to make sure she had locked up properly before she went to do her shopping.' She screwed up her eye

in another wink. 'She gets very worried in case somebody breaks in while she's away. She remembers a time
when thieves threatened her with all sorts of terrible
things unless she gave them a cup of tea and a biscuit.
Luckily she had just put the kettle on.'

I took the point of the two winks and in a round-
about way endeavoured, with Miss Macintosh, to
persuade Miss Silver that her post office days were
over and she had nothing to fear from nasty men with
guns. She was grateful for the assurance and insisted
on giving us both a small token of her gratitude. She
went to her flat and returned with a packet of Lincoln
Creams for me and a tin of shortbread for Miss
Macintosh.

Stew was the next to hint that Miss Silver should
have an eye kept on her as she seemed to be going
funny in the head. I reprimanded him for speaking so
disrespectfully of one of the residents but he was
unabashed. He was in my garden, whiling away time
when he should have been working. He stood on what
I optimistically called the lawn, hands in pockets and
chewing a blade of grass, watching me struggling to
remove a very large weed that seemed to have its roots
deep down in the earth's crust. He often did this,
ostensibly to give me a report on what he had done, or
more often, left undone. He and I both knew that the

true purpose of his visit was to have a chat with me, preferably over a cup of tea in my kitchen. I knew I should have been firm and instead of encouraging him in his laziness I should have reminded him of the odd jobs that were mounting up, waiting for him. But I lacked the necessary firmness to shift Stew when he was in the mood for talking.

He was a good talker if somewhat biased in his opinions on life, politics and God. Normally I kept off these topics but Stew always brought the conversation round to one or the other, and sometimes all three, depending on how long it took me to get rid of him.

He didn't go much on politics. I never knew whether he voted Labour, Liberal or Conservative. I had a sneaking suspicion that he put his cross against all three, because, as he said, it all came to much the same thing in the end. But he was constantly amazed that though politicians were only men like him they decided whether the world would be blown up or not. He didn't believe in all that war stuff, though he supposed if somebody pushed the button he would have to do his bit like everybody else.

Life, he said, was a funny thing when you came to think about it. He didn't think about it often because you'd go round the bend if you started trying to fathom what it was all in aid of. What got him, he said, was having to work when you ought to be enjoying yourself, seeing that life was so short.

He had been rather put out by the moon landings. He remembered being told at Sunday school that there was a home for little children above the clear blue sky, and believing it. But now he wasn't so sure. As a way of getting round the problem Stew tried to discount the landings: it was all one big con, he said, thought up by the Americans to fox the Russians. He almost talked me into believing that the men we had watched with bated breath hadn't been on the moon at all, but bouncing about on some enormous inflatable mattress.

I abandoned the weed and asked Stew if he would care for a cup of tea. He was in the kitchen before I got there.

'What makes you say that I ought to keep an eye on Miss Silver?' I asked him when he was sitting comfortably in the old armchair which my mother had brought with her when she came to spend her last few months with me.

'Well, it's your duty to keep an eye on them, isn't it?' he said rather saucily, helping himself to one of the Lincoln Creams that Miss Silver had given me. I ignored his tone. I felt there was something beneath it which had to be investigated.

'But why her in particular?' Stew took two more biscuits. 'She brought a chair down this morning and stood on it trying to get into Miss May's window.'

I tried not to laugh. Miss Silver was short and fat and had arthritic knees. It was difficult to imagine her climbing onto a chair, let alone easing herself through a window.

'It's nothing to laugh at,' said Stew sternly. 'If I hadn't been having a cup of tea with Mrs James when it happened she could have broken a leg or something and it would have taken me all week to mend it. It's the chair leg I'm talking about,' he added angrily, seeing me stifle another laugh. 'But it could have been *her* leg if she'd fallen off the chair. And what's more, if Miss May had caught sight of her trying to get in the window she'd have had a blue fit and been under the doctor for a month.'

The thought sobered me. Miss May had only just struggled to her feet after a week in bed. I was looking forward to a night or two of unbroken sleep. 'Where was I when all this was going on?' In my job as matron I was not only expected to be everywhere at once, but to have eyes in the back of my head. Failing to witness a resident trying to climb in another resident's window would go against me when the committee found out.

'You were where you usually are at that time in the morning,' said Stew. 'You were chasing up the street taking the prescriptions to Boots or queuing at the fish stall for a bit of halibut or something for somebody's dinner.' He and I both knew that the committee would have been reluctant to accept this as an excuse when I appeared before them at the inquisition.

'Did you ask her why she was doing it?'

'I did, but I couldn't make sense out of what she told me. She said she was looking for a policeman because there was a man in the post office helping himself to stamps. I told you she was going a bit funny in the head.'

I explained about the raid on the post office and his face saddened. 'Poor old girl,' he said, 'no wonder she's going barmy.' There was feeling in his voice. He was a kind-hearted young man.

I talked long and earnestly with Miss Silver and she nodded as if she perfectly understood what I was saying. I took her to the doctor and he gave her a prescription and told her to take the tablets three times a day after meals. If she felt no better after she had taken them all she was to go back to him for another lot. Since she didn't know that she was supposed to be ill, she was hardly likely to know when she was feeling better. It was left to me to see that she took the tablets and to watch for any change in her condition.

For a while things went smoothly. Miss Macintosh stopped following Miss Silver round the supermarket and Miss Silver appeared to have forgotten that she had once been a subpostmistress and been held at gunpoint by a wicked man. The tablets seemed to be working.

Then one day Stew came tearing up the garden path and burst in without knocking. He was in the same feverish state that Mrs Turgoose got into when she had a more than usually thrilling bit of gossip to impart.

'I thought you were supposed to be adjusting Miss Silver's ballcock,' I said coldly.

'It's her that I've come about,' he said. 'I bet you don't know what she's got in her drawers.'

I had to admit that except for the usual clutter which people keep in their drawers I couldn't have hazarded a guess.

'Well, I know,' he said. 'And the sooner you get across there and see for yourself, the better. And you might go through her cupboards as well while you're at it. You're in for a shock.' Like Mrs Turgoose, he could be tantalizingly mysterious at times.

I was reluctant to go but Stew was adamant. He even stood aside for me to go through the door first and didn't barge past me on the path. Then I knew the matter was urgent.

Miss Silver was delighted to see me. She spoke warmly of Stew, saying how efficiently he'd dealt with her ballcock. Then she said that as she was about to make some tea, maybe I would stay and have a cup. After she had poured the tea she went to the dresser, opened one of the cupboards and watched placidly as an avalanche of packets slid to the floor. From where I was sitting I saw Lincoln Creams, Rich Teas, Nice, Marie, fig rolls and digestives, chocolate and plain. In addition to the biscuits there were jam tarts in cellophane wrappers, little swiss rolls, slabs of family fruit cake and several packs of hot cross buns. It was autumn, so the buns must have been stale.

'Dear me,' said Miss Silver, 'I seem to have run out of ginger snaps.' She opened another cupboard and fought through the second avalanche. Failing to find any ginger snaps, she went through the dresser drawers flinging Peak Freans, McVities, Crawfords and Huntley & Palmers to right and left. When the search for the ginger snaps proved fruitless she went into the kitchen, with me close behind. She dived into a large cardboard box where the overspill was obviously kept, and came up with the ginger snaps in one hand and a cocoa tin in the other. The tin sparkled with tinsel. Fat, jolly Santa Clauses and bright red holly berries gave it a Yuletide look. A slot large enough for a coin to be pushed through had been cut out of the front. Above the slot were the words: 'Staff Xmas Box – Thank you.'

'Now how on earth could that have got there?' Miss Silver held up the tin and examined it closely. 'I must have bought it to give somebody for Christmas and then forgotten it. How silly of me.'

I took the tin off her and shook it. There was a very little rattle from the few coins it contained and I was relieved to know that it must have been removed from a counter, with other of Miss Silver's acquisitions, before the grateful staff had been given too many Christmas offerings by their satisfied customers. As another Christmas was well on its way I didn't think there was any need for me to go round the shops trying to establish who owned the tin.

I sent for the doctor and went to see the chairman of the committee. The doctor threw back his head and laughed uproariously when I opened the cupboards and drawers and showed him the collection of cakes and biscuits which Miss Silver had amassed since she came to the Lodge. I knew they weren't there when she arrived. I had helped her to unpack and would have noticed them. When the doctor had finished choking over the staff Christmas present tin he stepped up the tablets, added a few of another sort and begged me to let him know when the old lady started robbing banks. Being Irish he couldn't help seeing the funny side of things, and being particularly devoted to old ladies he was anxious to postpone the day when he would have to come to some decision about what he must do next to solve her problem – and mine as well.

The chairman of the committee was not amused. Like me, he foresaw all that might happen if Miss Silver went on confiscating things from the supermarket and was eventually caught. But he, like the doctor, had no wish to cause her any unhappiness. He said that he would put it on the agenda for the next meeting and meanwhile he trusted that I would do all in my power to stop her from bringing disgrace to the Lodge.

It was the day after I had spoken to the chairman, and before I'd had time to put Miss Silver under surveillance, that the telephone rang and the manager of the supermarket asked me if I would kindly get up there as quickly as I could. I hurried into the town, praying that there wouldn't be a police car parked outside the supermarket. There wasn't.

Miss Silver, the manager, and a nice young woman who said she was the store detective were seated at a table in the manager's office. On the table were one or two wrapped cakes, a packet of pretty pink wafer biscuits, a tin of sugared almonds and a giant box of liquorice allsorts. The allsorts box was open and I noticed a little black dribble running down Miss Silver's chin. I knew that the time had come when something decisive would have to be done.

It was a story quickly told. The young woman had caught Miss Silver in the act of stuffing cakes and biscuits into her shopping bag. When she walked past the checkout and into the street the young woman had touched her on the arm and asked her if she would like to step into the manager's office. Miss Silver said she would be delighted and on the way there she had stretched over and taken another cake down from a shelf. When questioned she offered the manager and the detective a liquorice allsort, which they took, being now almost as confused as she was. She explained that she liked to have plenty of cake in the house, and biscuits as well, in case somebody with a gun dropped in for a cup of tea. It was at this point that the manager rang for me. Miss Silver hadn't hesitated when they asked her where she lived. She seemed quite surprised that they didn't know.

'What are you going to do about her?' the manager asked when I described the incident that had triggered off Miss Silver's obsession. 'By rights I should be sending for the police but it hardly seems worth it with her mind the state it's in. Take her home and see that she never comes in here again.'

A very worried Miss Macintosh met us on the forecourt. She had seen Miss Silver go out but she hadn't known about the things I had found in Miss Silver's cupboards and drawers and had thought it was still safe to let her go to the shops alone.

'Whatever will become of her?' she asked, kind eyes brimming with tears. I told her not to worry, I would think of something, but in the end it was Stew who put his thinking cap on and came up with a solution.

'Didn't you tell me she'd got a nephew somewhere?' he said, when I was pouring out my troubles in his workshop. I did this sometimes, working on the assumption that two heads were better than one, especially if the one had run out of ideas. 'Why don't you write to him, tell him what's happened and see if he'll have her? She'd probably be a different woman if she was with somebody all the time.'

I said that I didn't think it would do much good. The nephew hardly ever came to see her and he had flatly refused to have her live with him and his new wife after his uncle died.

'That was then,' said Stew. 'People change, you know. I should think he'd rather she went to live with them than have to go to that place up the road.' He meant the new psychiatric hospital that had lately been built. 'It wouldn't do any harm to write to him. You could even give him a ring. His number's bound to be in her records, him being next of kin.'

I gave the nephew a ring and he came at once. He seemed quite cross that I hadn't sent for him sooner.

'If you'd let me know she was going funny in the head she could have come and lived with us and maybe none of this would have happened.' I got the impression that he was blaming me for everything.

'But I thought you said it wasn't convenient for you to have your aunt living with you,' I said a trifle indignantly. I remembered how adamant he'd been about it.

'Yes well, but things were different then. We'd only just got married and she wasn't going round nicking things from supermarkets. You can't have her locked up just for pinching biscuits. She was uncle's favourite sister and he'd turn in his ashes if he thought we weren't looking after her when she needed it. Besides, the wife's expecting. She'll be glad of a bit of help when the baby comes. Aunt's not too far gone for that, is she?'

I said that Miss Silver was quite capable of washing a few nappies, but he said they'd got a washing machine. What they might want, he said, was for her to rock the baby if it was crying when the wife was trying to get its bottle ready. I said I thought Miss Silver would be willing and able to do that. She might even be able to baby-sit occasionally so long as they made sure that the doors were locked and nobody could get in through the windows. He said there was no chance of that, he was a locksmith and the place was like Fort Knox. He suddenly seemed quite happy at the prospect of having his aunt to live with him.

'I told you people changed,' said Stew when I told him the outcome of the nephew's visit. 'I remember when my gran started to get a bit past it and she came to live with us. My dad hated it at first but he got over it and he was ever so cut up when she died. I used to like her living with us. She often slipped me sixpence to go to Saturday morning pictures, and she'd never let Dad hit me even if she knew I'd asked for it. She was a bit of all right, was my gran.'

Miss Macintosh was delighted by what had happened. 'There you are, you see,' she said. 'All's well that ends well. How nice for Miss Silver and what a pity it is that dear Miss Cromwell hasn't got a nephew or somebody to take her to live with them. We should sadly miss her, I know, but none of us would be so selfish as to wish to keep her here if she could be happy elsewhere.'

Chapter Ten

MISS MACINTOSH WASN'T the only one who dreamed of the day when some long-lost relatives would turn up from somewhere and take Miss Cromwell under their wing. Nor was it only the residents who dreamed the impossible dream. I had moments of fantasy when an emergency bell rang and I hurried across the forecourt, to be met by a rampaging Miss Cromwell and whichever of her neighbours she had chosen to upset that day.

I had made her acquaintance before she came to the Lodge. Hers had been one of the names on the Christmas list. She lived then in a small terraced house which, like so many others in the town, was demolished to make room for bigger if not better things. When the demolition was imminent her name was put forward to the committee, who delved into her past, satisfied themselves that it was blameless and allowed her name to go on the waiting list for a flat. And blameless her past had been, despite the reputation she had for a biting tongue, and her gift for making enemies. These were two of the little weaknesses which the committee seldom took into account when they were deciding who was eligible to come into the Lodge. They knew, being a charitable body, that women with either or both of the weaknesses were less likely to be taken under somebody's wing than their sweeter-natured sisters.

On the first occasion that I delivered the Christmas envelopes I was kept standing on the doorstep while Miss Cromwell examined the enclosure and signed the ledger with a flowing scrawl that took up all her own line and those above and below it. She slammed the ledger shut and handed it back to me without a word. But the Christmas before she moved into the Lodge, when she knew that her name was nearing the top of the list, she opened the door to its widest extent, invited me in and gave me two cups of very strong tea. I guessed that the warmth of her welcome was intended to pave the way for an equally warm welcome when she took up residence.

While I was drinking the tea I noticed that there were no family photographs hanging on her walls or adorning her mantelpiece. Instead, she had portraits of royalty everywhere. Kings and queens, princes and princesses stood or sat, singly or in groups. Victoria and Albert were much in evidence. With or without each other, they stared imperiously ahead, watching the birdie but defying the photographer to make them say anything as vulgar as cheese. Later, when Miss Cromwell moved to the Lodge, I was surprised to learn that she was against the monarchy, frequently expressing the opinion that the money spent on its upkeep should be put to a better purpose. But she still cut out pictures of the royal family when they appeared in the papers.

In all the years that I knew her she never looked any different. She charged through the streets and in and out of the shops, round hat bobbling with every step she took. Her black, sensible lace-up shoes could have been army issue from their size and the brilliance of their polish. She could have been army issue herself with her ramrod back, stentorian voice and brisk manly stride. Even when she wasn't in her outdoor clothes the severity of her blouses and skirts managed to convey the impression that she was wearing uniform. This added to the confusion she caused when she arrived at the Lodge and began thinking that she was the matron.

But for all her forbidding image and the difficulty she had in maintaining good relations with her neighbours, Miss Cromwell was a staunch supporter of worthy causes. Whenever there was a flag or a poppy to be sold she could be found standing on draughty street corners, or sheltering in doorways, rattling her tin and intimidating passers-by with her menacing glare. She rattled and glared to such good purpose that those she accosted took fright and dropped more in her tin than they had intended. Miss Cromwell paid no regard to the ruling that nobody should be bullied or coerced into parting with their money. She was much sought after as a flag seller.

As well as standing with trays full of emblems and pins she marched round the pubs on Saturday nights threatening the customers with hell fire unless they renounced the demon drink and went home to their wives, or whoever was waiting for them there. Some were so shaken by the picture she drew of purgatory that they downed their pints and ordered another to give them the courage to face it.

Even before I started delivering the annual Christmas present to Miss Cromwell I knew her well by sight. I had encountered her in the town, carving a path through the crowds that thronged the market at weekends. I had nervously shrunk from her in the shops, and waited behind her in the queue while she worked out how much she thought her bill should be and checked the result with the amount the girl on the till had charged her. The two sums never tallied and the girl on the till either got so overwrought that she burst into tears and conceded to Miss Cromwell or she stuck to her guns and sent for the manager.

Those in the queue started by exchanging sympathetic glances and speaking in defence of poor old ladies who couldn't stand up for themselves and were short-changed by shop girls and others intent on doing them out of their rights. But as time slipped by the mood of the queue got ugly. People changed sides and started muttering about poor young shop assistants who were constantly being put on by bad-tempered customers. Unlike the sympathetic championing, the mutterings were too low to reach Miss Cromwell's ears, and if she had heard them she would have stood her ground. She knew she was right, even after the manager had proved beyond all reasonable doubt that she wasn't.

The flat which became empty to allow Miss Cromwell to move in was at the opposite end of the verandah from Mrs Peters. I was glad of this. Remembering the delays that both of them could cause in queues, and the way both of them elbowed others when they were trying to get to a stall in the market, the thought of them being next-door neighbours would have kept me awake at nights. The occasional breach of the peace I could cope with but inviting more by putting two residents with the same quick temper close to one another was something to be avoided. It had happened once and for a while the Lodge had resounded with angry choruses while Mrs Peters and Mrs Mundy – stepping from the adjacent doors – aired their differences at the top of their voices.

Mrs Mundy had been admitted on a temporary basis while her family made their final arrangements for emigrating and taking her with them. When I mentioned to Mrs Turgoose that I was putting her next to Mrs Peters she had given me warning of what would happen.

'You'll live to regret it,' she said. 'You're asking for trouble if you put those two within ten flats of each other. They're both nasty-tempered and the sparks'll fly the minute they cross each other's paths, which they'll have to do often if they're living next door to one another.'

'I wish you wouldn't interfere,' I told her crossly. 'I've got nowhere else to put her and for all you know they could get on like a house on fire.' I was already beginning to doubt it. Mrs Turgoose was pretty reliable with her warnings and if she said sparks would fly there was every chance that they would.

'Have it your own way but don't say I didn't warn you,' she said. 'After all, you're the matron. All I'm saying is I know Mundy and I know Peters and I've seen sparks flying when they get together at the Sunshine Club. It's murder when they're enjoying a game of cards together, or sitting next to each other when we're playing bingo. The warden often has to separate them.'

Mrs Peters had been very put out when I told her who was moving into the flat next to hers. That it was only on a temporary basis did nothing to appease her. If anything, it roused her to further anger.

'That woman's got no right to come in here,' she snarled. 'This isn't a holiday camp, it's a place where people live. And if I know Ella Mundy she'll cause as much trouble here as she does everywhere else. She gets the pick of everything down at the Club. Even when she has her dinner there she somehow manages to get bigger helpings than everybody else. I shouldn't wonder if it wasn't a put-up job between her and them as serves them out. Mind you, I got my own back on her once. I leaned across for the salt and accidently tipped a plateful of red-hot soup in her lap. It was a scream. The soup went right through her frock. We didn't see her down there for a week or two and when she came back she got quite huffy when we asked her to show us the scalds. They were in an awkward place, I shouldn't wonder.' Mrs Peters smiled happily at the memory.

Mrs Mundy wasn't pleased either when she learned who was to be her neighbour until the time came for her to emigrate. The affair of the soup still rankled.

'It beats me how she ever got in here,' she said when she was running down Mrs Peters. 'We all know she's got some premium bonds, and I for one have stood behind her in the post office and seen how much she's been putting away. I was always given to understand that this place was for those who haven't got anything, not for people like her with premium bonds.'

The first time the two ladies drew swords emergency bells rang, pigeons fell over each other in their haste to get away and the ginger cat, which was still in residence at the time, went off and didn't return for a week.

'There, what did I tell you?' cried Mrs Turgoose triumphantly. 'I warned you what it would be like if those two were put within shouting distance of each other. I should have thought you'd have been here long enough by now to know better than to walk into trouble with your eyes wide open.'

I maintained a dignified silence. There were times

when I knew that Mrs Turgoose was right but I seldom gave her the satisfaction of hearing me admit it.

When Miss Cromwell first came in it had been an embarrassment having to explain to those who didn't know that the lady who stumped along the verandah in her professional-looking clothes was a resident and not the matron. Not only were scouts deceived into removing the railings, and workmen sent away before they had done what they came to do, but new doctors visiting the Lodge for the first time were equally deceived. A nervous young man who called to see Mrs James when she had a rash on her chest went away looking vastly relieved that he was only standing in for the regular doctor and wouldn't have to call too often. The experience left him shaken.

He had been met on the verandah by Miss Cromwell in full sail, and in full dress. She was carrying the little black bag she had bought to make her job as matron easier. Taking it for granted that she was who she said she was he followed respectfully, two paces behind the majestic lady. Unfortunately she had misheard him when he told her who he had come to see, and instead of leading him to Mrs James's flat she took him to see Miss May. Miss Macintosh, who was standing at her window while Miss Cromwell and the doctor were getting to know each other, saw what was happening and rang her bell for me. I got across just in time to save Miss May from having to bare her chest to a man who was not only a stranger but a foreigner to boot. None of her doctors had been foreign.

The Asian doctor, with a less than perfect command of his second language, looked quite distraught when I got there. And so did Miss May. She sat up in bed clutching at shawls while Miss Cromwell, perfectly in control of the situation, stood stiff and straight, a tablespoon in one hand and a notebook and pencil in the other, the epitome of professionalism.

'Darling matron,' cried Miss May when she saw me. She reached out and grabbed my hand. 'Oh, darling matron, I'm so glad you're here. I keep trying to tell the doctor that I'm not under him, but Miss Cromwell says I am. She wants me to show him my chest but it's quite out of the question since I don't even know who he is.' She laid her head on the pillows, too shocked to say any more. The doctor stood bemused, no doubt wondering what the BMA would make of it all when he appeared before them accused of whatever they would find him guilty of doing.

I coaxed Miss Cromwell out of the room and gave Miss May a few sips of brandy. Then I turned my attention to the doctor, who looked as if he could have done with the brandy himself if his religion didn't forbid it. I tried to explain that there had been a break-down of communications somewhere along the verandah and it was Mrs James's chest he should have been examining and not Miss May's. Though I spoke very slowly and in a loud voice there were still things that he didn't understand.

'But if you are the matron, then who is the lady who has just left the room?' He patted Miss May's hand to let her know that she was in no way to blame for the mix-up, whereupon she siezed his hand and kissed it. After that she would have been quite happy to let him look at her chest, but I stopped her unfastening her nightdress and told her to take a nap instead.

'Oh, that was just a resident who thinks she's the matron,' I said, trying to sound as if it was the most natural thing in the world for residents to go round thinking they were matrons. He still looked puzzled.

'But why did she bring me here instead of taking me to where I should have been?' He had started to get slightly irritated by what he took to be the inscrutable ways of English ladies.

'She's a bit deaf,' I lied, 'she didn't hear you prop-erly.' It would have taken too long to explain that not many Asian doctors came to the Lodge, and the mistake had arisen from the language problem. He followed me to Mrs James's flat and cast some very curious looks in my direction while he examined her chest.

The rash was diagnosed as an allergy caused by Mrs James handling the tomato plants which the old gardener gave to her to fill up a corner in the south side of her little garden. It cleared up quickly after she had applied the cream which the doctor ordered. The old gardener took the tomato plants away and replaced them with marrows. He gave Mrs James detailed instructions on how to fertilize them by doing some rather intimate things with a rabbit's foot. Mrs James fluttered her eyelashes when she was telling me this. I don't think she ever got the hang of cross-pollination. Her marrows came to nothing.

I didn't take Miss Cromwell to task for allowing the doctor to think she was the matron; we were all used to it by then. Neither did I upbraid her for taking him to see Miss May instead of Mrs James. I knew how easy it was for such errors to arise when two people of different origins were trying to make themselves understood. There had been many such errors made when immigrants started arriving in numbers. Forenames were confused with surnames and none of the names were easy to pronounce. It was as hard for us as it was for them. Miss Cromwell could be forgiven for thinking the doctor had said Miss May and not Mrs James.

It was after Miss Cromwell had rung the Gas Board in her role as matron and ordered twenty new cookers that I thought the time had come to have a word with her own GP. Though she was on his panel he didn't know her, except from seeing her around the town.

'Miss Cromwell thinks she's the matron,' I said, when I caught him as he was going to visit somebody else. She had her own cures for minor ills and never needed a doctor.

'Well?' he queried, waiting for more.

'She stops the workmen and tells them to go away, and last week she ordered twenty new cookers from the Gas Board.'

It was the Irish doctor, the one who had been convulsed at the thought of Miss Silver stocking her cupboards with assorted biscuits. He could hardly control himself at the thought of Miss Cromwell ordering twenty cookers from the Gas Board.

'Did they deliver them?' he spluttered.

'No, but they might have done if she hadn't been in the week before and ordered twenty refrigerators. Luckily there's a six-week wait and somebody in the shop recognized Miss Cromwell and knew she wasn't the matron.'

'Then there's nothing for you to worry about,' he said, climbing into his shabby old car. 'Let me know when she starts thinking she's the doctor and I'll see what we can do about it.' He drove off, singing at the top of his voice.

Chapter Eleven

THERE WERE MURMURINGS amongst the residents when Mrs Koloski reached the top of the list and moved into the flat next to Mrs Dean. Mrs Koloski was the woman who had been expected sooner. It was she who had kept the betting shop and had ulcerated legs, and though it had been established by the committee before she came in that the business had been run on perfectly respectable lines, and not a breath of scandal had touched the proprietress, there were those round the Lodge who were not over-anxious to welcome her into their midst. I heard the murmurings when I did the rounds.

'Oh dear, surely not her,' said Mrs Dean, when I told her who her new neighbour was going to be. Then, realizing that she had sounded uncharitable, she went on quickly, 'It's not that I've got anything against her personally and I'd be the last person in the world to condemn a woman for keeping a betting shop.

Everyone to their taste, as they say in France, but this isn't France and I can't think of anything that would be further from my taste.'

'Did you know her when she kept the betting shop?' I asked.

'Naturally I didn't know her,' replied Mrs Dean, with an edge to her voice. 'But I used to see her through the window when I did my shopping. She had ulcerated legs, if my memory serves me right, and always sat with her feet up. I was civil, of course, and nodded when I passed, but that's not quite the same as having her for a next-door neighbour.' She snapped her mouth shut in a tight line, then opened it again. 'I've always had standards and I've never approved of gambling in any shape or form. She and I will have absolutely nothing in common.'

Mrs Dean had lived for a long time with the misconception that she was responsible for her daughter's death. She remained convinced that had she not weakened and given her consent to the marriage, the car crash wouldn't have happened and they would still be living cosily in the house near the park. Family and friends had done all they could to make her think otherwise but to no avail. In the end her doctor had told them to stop trying. Far better, he said, to let her think what she wanted to think rather than keep upsetting her by arguing. Reluctantly, they took his advice. She was much happier then, and accepted her guilt as a cross she had to bear, visiting the cemetery several times a week and spending more than she could afford on flowers. She never took flowers to her son-in-law's grave. Though she had grown fond of him as time passed, after her daughter was killed she preferred to think he had never existed.

Miss Macintosh was another who wasn't overjoyed at the thought of Mrs Koloski coming in. She put down her sewing when I told her and picked nervously at her pinafore.

'That wouldn't be the woman who kept the betting shop on the High Street?' she asked when I mentioned the rather unusual name. I confirmed that it was and she sat nervously nibbling her lower lip.

I couldn't help wondering why Miss Macintosh should be so concerned at Mrs Koloski coming in. I knew she had standards – she was a very upright woman – but she wasn't the sort to impose them on others. I remember her telling me that it was all right having standards so long as you lived up to them your-self and didn't expect everybody else to do the same. I didn't think she could be nibbling her lip because of the betting shop. She wasn't averse to having a flutter when I took a basin round on Grand National day, inviting the residents to pick a horse in return for sixpence. Miss Macintosh always had two dips into the basin, and would have had more but for a streak of native caution.

'Do you know the woman who's coming in?' I asked her. She fidgeted with a loose thread that was dangling at the front of her cardigan.

'I used to,' she said, giving the thread a sharp tug which caused a button to fall off the cardigan. 'I knew her years ago before her husband died. That's why I'm so worried about her coming in here.' She rummaged through her sewing basket until she found some thread that matched her cardigan. While she was sewing the button back on I got her to tell me what was so worrying about Mrs Koloski coming in.

'The office I worked in was next door to the shop and I used to go in sometimes and put sixpence each way on a horse. Once or twice I even went as far as risking a shilling. But that was only when there was a big race. I'm terrified in case she recognizes me and points me out to Mrs Turgoose or any of the others. It would be all round the place in minutes. I could never look anybody in the face again.' She flushed hotly at the thought of the good reputation she had (despite some of the residents still believing she was an heiress) being torn to shreds by an indiscreet disclosure about her past.

'I took after my father, I'm afraid. He was a gambler. I expect I had it in my blood. But I hated walking into the betting shop with all those men lounging about, swearing and smelling of beer and tobacco.' She shuddered at the thought.

'Did you ever win anything?' I asked, to take her mind off the smelly men in the betting shop. She shook her head.

'Never,' she said. 'I took after my father for that as well. He was a good man but he often came home on Fridays without any wages. Mother did dressmaking to pay for my typing lessons, which was one of the reasons why I never married. I felt that I owed it to her to stay at home after father died, to pay her back for the sacrifices she made for me.' I had heard that story many times before from spinster ladies round the Lodge.

'I think I was bitten by the gambling bug at an early age,' said Miss Macintosh, after a moment's quietness. 'I could never resist the slot machines on the pier, even when I went with the Sunday school outing, and later it got even worse. I always used to buy a whole book of raffle tickets instead of just one when they were brought round the office at Christmas. I never won anything on those either. The awful thing is that I've often been tempted to go to bingo at that place in the

High Street that used to be a cinema. The only thing that's kept me away is the thought of somebody who knows me seeing me in the queue waiting to get in.'

She sounded so ashamed of herself that I drew up my chair close to hers and did what I could to ease her conscience. I told her how I was never able to tear myself away from the slot machines on the pier when I went to the seaside for my holidays. I put in penny after penny, then stood mesmerized watching lemons, blackcurrants and other fruits whizzing round until they slowed down and stopped. On the rare occasions that the fruit came to rest in a winning order I ploughed back the winnings, and much more besides, until I had far exceeded my spending allowance for the day. I confessed that I also bought whole books of raffle tickets in the vain hope of carrying off a Christmas hamper or the £50 top prize. I further bared my soul, in an attempt to show her that she wasn't the only one with weaknesses, and admitted that though I didn't go into betting shops because I didn't like the atmosphere, I had often given Stew a shilling to put on a horse which he had told me couldn't possibly be beaten. She was heartened to hear that I had never once got my shilling back.

After she had thanked me for not condemning her for her addiction to gambling I thought of something else. I reminded her that she was a good deal older than when she worked in the office and it was unlikely that Mrs Koloski would know her again. 'Furthermore,' I said, 'I wouldn't be surprised if there isn't a code amongst bookmakers, as there is with doctors, lawyers and other professional people, which makes it unethical for them to talk about their clients.' This cheered her immensely.

Miss May remembered Mrs Koloski well. They had often shared an ambulance and had sat together in out-patients' when Mrs Koloski was going up to the hospital with her legs, and Miss May with whatever she was under the doctor for at the time. 'Of course, she was never as bad as I was,' said Miss May, jealously guarding her right to suffer more than most. 'And as far as I remember, her legs got better.' She said this as if in some way it was a reflection on Mrs Koloski.

Mrs Turgoose told me again all she had told me before about the incoming resident, adding that somebody at the Darby and Joan club had said she used to be a Miss Green before she married the man with the Russian-sounding name.

'It seems funny him having a name like one of them Russkies,' she said.

'Perhaps he was a Russian,' I said. 'Perhaps he was

one of those Russians with the dancing bears that you told the reporter about when he came to interview you after you spread it around the town that you'd won a fortune on the Irish Sweep.' She ignored the allusion to one of her past follies.

'No, Ivy Koloski's husband wasn't a Russian. He was one of the evacuees who came down here when Jerry was bombing London. A lot of them had funny names. As far as I can understand, London's crawling with people with funny names who can't speak proper English.'

Mrs Koloski spoke perfect English. She was an inch or two shorter than Miss Cromwell, but as powerfully built. She had a great deal of black, frizzy hair, and a purplish face which I thought indicated a heart condition, but which she said she'd inherited from her grandfather. She, like Miss Cromwell, wore clothes that were starkly severe; she had very large feet. Her legs broke down occasionally but, as Miss May had said, they were vastly improved since the days when she sat in the betting shop with them up on a chair.

But though there were similarities between Miss Cromwell and the new resident, they were very different in temperament. Mrs Koloski was a mild-mannered woman, friendly with everybody even if they were unfriendly towards her. It wasn't long before some of her neighbours were calling her Ivy, and talking to her as if she had never owned a betting shop. She showed her appreciation by doing little kindnesses, such as bringing in shopping for somebody who had a cold and was nursing it. She helped Mrs James to propagate her pansies and spread compost over the barren marrows. She dropped in often to have a nice little chat with Miss May, and wasn't above bringing in a scuttle of coal if the home help hadn't turned up or had forgotten to do it. Miss May was the last at the Lodge to use solid fuel. The central heating at full blast was but background heat for her.

When Miss Macintosh tripped over a slip mat and turned her ankle Mrs Koloski, hanging heavily on to the banister, climbed upstairs several times a day to make her a cup of tea. If she recognized the woman who had lost heavily on the horses she gave no sign of it, and gradually the worry lines on Miss Macintosh's brow disappeared. There was something about Ivy Koloski that made it hard not to like her. Even Mrs Dean was heard to say, albeit grudgingly, that though she wasn't exactly a lady she had a lot of good points.

Mrs Peters was one of the last to respond to Ivy's friendly overtures. She kept her standing at the door when she went across to ask if Mrs Peters would care to come over to her place for a cup of tea. Nobody had ever asked Mrs Peters such a thing before. She was so taken aback that she shut the door without saying a word, leaving Ivy standing on the step wondering what she'd done wrong.

'It's the name she doesn't like,' said Mrs Turgoose when she was telling me about the reception Ivy got from Mrs Peters. 'Mrs Peters can't stand people with foreign names. She can't stand foreigners either. She says it stands to reason they have to think in English so why they have to go round jabbering in a language nobody can make head or tail of is beyond her. I don't mind telling you that it's beyond me as well.'

But in spite of her aversion to Mrs Koloski's name, even Mrs Peters couldn't fail to unbend when Ivy offered to peg out her washing when she'd got a touch of bronchitis and the wind was in the east. To everybody's surprise she started wandering along the verandah on warm days, sat on the bench with Ivy and one or two others, and talked of the time when the High Street wasn't cluttered with supermarkets and shops with music blaring out all day. As soon as Miss Macintosh's ankle had mended sufficiently for her to get down the stairs she became part of the group, adding a Scottish flavour to the Sassenach fun. Eventually Stew had to bring an extra bench from the garden to provide seats for all those who made the most of the summer days and sat listening to Ivy telling them about life in a betting shop. Mrs Dean peeped wistfully out of her window until one afternoon she took her first faltering steps to become part of the happy gathering. She frowned when Mrs Turgoose got carried away and said something suggestive, but Ivy quickly gave Mrs Turgoose a dig in the ribs and told her to mind her manners. Poor Mrs Turgoose had sore ribs for a long time.

Only Miss Cromwell stayed aloof. Sometimes she hovered near the benches, pretending to be looking into the gully to check if Stew had cleaned it properly. When she walked away it was noticeable that she didn't stride out as briskly as usual. And she didn't bang her door as she had done before. There was something about the packed benches and the laughter of the residents that seemed to deter her from making her presence felt in an aggressive way.

She also thought twice before she ground her heels into Mrs James's garden when Ivy was helping to thin out the seedlings. For a while after Stew had chalked up the notice warning trespassers that the garden was private, Miss Cromwell had given it a fairly wide berth. But after the chalk began to be washed off by the winter rains she started drawing in closer until once again she was leaving her heel marks in the borders which Mrs James kept knife-edged with a long pair of clippers that the gardener had lent her. The heel marks got deeper and deeper and further in, until they eroded the blue lobelia and snowy alyssum. I had begun to dread the day when Mrs James, with tears in her eyes, would beg me to do my matronly duty and remind Miss Cromwell that she was trampling not only on Mrs James's garden but on her feelings. Suddenly it began to seem as if I was to be spared the trouble.

The next surprise in store for everybody came when Miss Cromwell asked me in when I did the round one morning. The news spread like wildfire and when I came out of her flat Mrs Turgoose and one or two others were waiting for me. I swept past them, giving them no time to comment on the event that had brought them there. It was common knowledge that even though I was the matron I had never been allowed in her flat since the day she moved in.

I had only time to notice that everywhere was in apple-pie order before she told me what I was there for.

'Who's that new woman that's come in?' she asked, pulling aside her nets and glancing through the window in the direction of the benches, where Ivy was already sitting, taking the morning air with Miss Macintosh.

'It's Mrs Koloski,' I replied, 'I expect you remember her. She used to keep a betting shop in the High Street.'

Miss Cromwell nodded thoughtfully. The little round hat and the black bag were on a small table, underneath which were her gleaming shoes. Her military style coat and severe jacket hung in a recess with the plastic raincoat she wore when she went out in the rain. The skirt she had on looked as if it had been freshly pressed and her white blouse had the pristine appearance of the newly washed.

'I thought it was her,' Miss Cromwell said, looking out again at the bench. 'I used to see her in the shop when I went on Saturdays to watch the football match. I saw her at the match once, but that was before her husband died and she took over the business.' She said no more and I realized that it was time for me to go. She shut the door behind me, but very quietly.

When I mentioned to Miss Macintosh that Miss Cromwell didn't storm up and down the verandah as much as she had once done, and nobody rang their bell to complain that she was going out of her way to annoy them, Miss Macintosh gave the matter some consideration and offered an explanation.

'Do you suppose it's got something to do with Ivy?'

she asked. I stared at her. The thought had crossed my mind but I'd dismissed it as nonsense.

'But why should it have anything to do with Ivy? They never speak to each other and Miss Cromwell still waits, as she's always done, until everybody's gone in before she comes out and sits on the verandah.'

'I know all about that,' said Miss Macintosh, 'but it still seems strange that she should have become so much less aggressive since Ivy moved in. And I've seen her once or twice when we've been out there, pretending to look in the gully as if she was plucking up courage to join us.'

It was hard to imagine her doing anything like that. Almost as soon as she came to the Lodge she had used the verandah as a lookout post. She had sat in the porch, which in those days was empty except for the hanging baskets, keeping an eagle eye on the comings and goings on the forecourt. Whenever a car came up the cul-de-sac and looked as if it intended to stay, Miss Cromwell was across the grass like a flash, ready to interrogate the driver. Unless they were regular visitors, or could prove that they were authorized to park, she terrified them into reversing sharply and going out the way they had come. Even those who had a perfect right to park under a copper beech, or against a pigeon-splattered wall, were at first deceived into thinking that a new rule had come into force since they last visited their aged relative.

Suddenly Miss Macintosh's words came true. Stew dashed across to me full of excitement at the latest development. He also had been watching Miss Cromwell, and had noticed the change in her.

'Here, guess what!' he exclaimed, and gave me no time to guess. 'It's Miss Cromwell. She's sitting on the verandah talking to Mrs Koloski.' If I didn't believe him, he said, all I had to do was walk up my path, out of my gate and see for myself. I believed him but I still had to see for myself.

The two women were sitting in the porch, heads together, apparently sharing a newspaper.

'There, what did I tell you?' said Stew after I had shut the gate, scarcely able to believe what I'd seen. 'They've been like that for ages but I haven't managed to find out what they're doing.'

I wanted to say 'then go and out find out', but being matron I couldn't.

'I'll go and clean out the gully again,' said Stew. 'Maybe if I got a bit closer to them I could look over their shoulders.' He was gone and back again in less than no time.

'They're doing the pools,' he gasped. 'They've got today's paper and a coupon and they're doing the pools.'

I knew he couldn't have been mistaken. He did the pools regularly, living in hopes that come Saturday when the results were read out he would be a rich man. When I asked him what he would do with his riches, should he ever get eight draws, he didn't hesitate. Unlike some pools winners who declare that their lives would be unaffected by having half a million pounds in the bank, Stew's eyes lit up at the thought of being able to part-exchange his very old banger for something rather less ancient. Beyond that he appeared to have no plans for disposing of half a million.

'Did you know that Miss Cromwell had started going into Ivy Koloski's place on Saturday afternoons?' Mrs Turgoose asked me one day. I didn't know. I had been so overtaken by the events of the past few weeks – Miss Cromwell asking me in when I did the rounds, sitting in the porch with the others, and nobody ringing her bell to complain about her – that I hadn't noticed that on top of all this she was going into Ivy's place on Saturday afternoons.

'She goes in there regular round about four,' said Mrs Turgoose. 'I shouldn't 'alf like to know what they get up to every week.' She nudged me and winked. 'It strikes me they've got a couple of blokes in there.' I gave her a cold look and left her before she became too inventive about the goings-on in Mrs Koloski's flat on Saturday afternoons.

It was round about four o'clock one Saturday that Mrs Koloski's son rang me and asked if I'd mind going across to tell his mother, who wasn't yet on the phone, that he would be picking her up as usual on Sunday for lunch. I said that I would go at once and tell her.

I had to knock several times, and very loudly, before Ivy opened the door. The living room was in darkness except for the flickering light from the television set. On the screen two large sweating men were grappling together, biceps straining and bald heads glistening. Grunts and groans came from the depths of their knotted throats. I saw Miss Cromwell sitting on the edge of her chair, too absorbed in the wrestling to have noticed me.

'You'd better sit down for a minute,' whispered Mrs Koloski. 'It's nearly the end of the round and it only needs a knockout to decide the winner.'

I groped my way round the room until I found a chair. At that moment one of the wrestlers fell to the canvas with an enormous thump. Miss Cromwell stood up and began to count, a bell rang and the victorious giant gave his writhing opponent a final contemptuous kick. Mrs Koloski turned on the light and Miss Cromwell sank back in her chair. She looked quite wrung out with the excitement of watching the wrestling.

'Cor blimey,' exclaimed Mrs Koloski, 'that was the best bout we've seen in weeks. Them heavyweights are worth watching. I like a bit of muscle myself. I can't stand it when you get a couple of chaps as light as feathers, ballet dancing round the ring.' She picked up two sixpences that were on the table and put them in her purse. 'Miss Cromwell and me always have a little flutter on Saturdays. This week it was her bloke that hit the canvas.' She smiled in commiseration at the loser. 'But she won last week so it evens things up. She's coming in later to watch the football and as it's Spurs playing Arsenal I expect we shall put a bit on. I support Spurs myself but she favours Arsenal to win.'

'You were right for once,' I told Mrs Turgoose the next time I saw her. 'Miss Cromwell and Ivy do have a couple of men in on Saturday afternoons.' I left her with her mouth open, already putting on her shawl to go and spread rumours round the Lodge.

Never again did Miss Cromwell march up and down the verandah watching for somebody to break rules she had once made to suit herself. She hadn't time. Throughout the cricket season she sat glued to her friend's television set, cheering loudly when the player she had set her hopes on made his century, and booing when the hapless wicket keeper let a ball go past. In the winter she urged on both teams to put the boot in. And when they weren't watching football or cricket the ladies sat willing their horses to clear the fences and gallop down the straight to the winning post. The highlights of their lives were the contests for the heavyweight boxing titles.

Soon, others around the Lodge were getting involved in sport, though not with quite the enthusiasm of Miss Cromwell and Ivy. Ladies who previously had only watched tennis sat in the porch, their daily papers turned to the back pages, reading the racing results or checking their pools coupons. Ivy went round showing them where to put the crosses and explaining the intricacies of an each-way bet. Mrs Peters, who, it turned out, had been doing the pools for years, but in secret, won a fourth dividend the first time she tried the system that Stew's dad had been using with no success since the day he was demobbed. The dividend was very small but it encouraged others to fill in football coupons. A new spirit came over the Lodge. Saturday night took on a new meaning with everybody gathered round their radios or television sets to hear the results.

Inevitably, the gambling fever spread. Mrs Turgoose raffled a bunch of plastic flowers, the proceeds to go to her favourite charity. Nobody ever found out which was her favourite charity but Miss Cromwell won the flowers and the next time I went into her flat I saw she had placed them beside a picture of Queen Victoria in mourning for her dearest Albert.

The news that Miss Cromwell was no longer a gorgon spread through the town. Shop girls who had once fallen over each other to get out of her way now fell over each other to serve her. People in queues insisted on her preceding them in the slow move forward. But her collecting tins were never as full on flag days. She had lost the menacing look which had persuaded people to give generously.

Chapter Twelve

Ivy was a godsend to me. She was a godsend to everybody round the Lodge. She was always ready to lend a hand if she thought she was needed, and she was the first to hear a cry for help and go to the rescue, though not always in the way that anybody expected.

When the old gardener finally retired and could no longer even ride his bike to come and visit Mrs James she would most certainly have reverted to the unhappy state she was in when she arrived at the Lodge if Ivy hadn't been there to cheer her up. She missed him dropping in and sharing her supper, and browsing through seed catalogues with her.

But Ivy refused to let her sink back into a lonely dreariness. When the weather was fine she made her put on her hat and coat and the two of them would use their old age pension bus passes to visit a garden centre that wasn't far from the Lodge. The people at the centre soon got used to seeing the two women, one with her legs bandaged, the other leaning on the stick she had used since her rheumatism got worse. They couldn't afford to buy much but they spent whole mornings or afternoons walking slowly between rows of brightly coloured bedding plants, pots of flowering shrubs and tubs of dwarf conifers, or the varieties that would grow to a great height if they didn't die off before they were firmly established. The garden centre was noted for its gnomes and Ivy and Mrs James made friends with Snow White and the seven dwarfs, pixies sitting on mushrooms, and little gnome fishermen. Naming the dwarfs was easy but they changed the pixies' and fishermen's names almost every time they went.

After they had paid a visit to the garden centre they sat on the verandah and blinded the residents with the science of gardening. They used Latin names (pronounced wrongly) for simple English flowers, and talked glibly of growing media when all they meant was a few rotted cabbage leaves and the little heaps of manure that Ivy scooped off the forecourt after a rag and bone man had been round, raucously calling for things to fill his cart.

One or two of the residents turned up their noses in disgust when they saw what the horse had left behind on the forecourt. But not so Ivy. It hardly had time to cool before she was rushing out with pan and brush getting it together for Mrs James's garden. 'Waste not, want not,' she cried joyously, spreading the growing medium lavishly along rows of weakly plants. In spite of the treatment many of them still died.

Ivy's talent for making others happy went far beyond collecting horse manure, visiting garden centres and showing people how to fill in their football coupons. She had skills which were only revealed after she had lived at the Lodge for a fair length of time. Miss May was the first to tell me that she could see the future in the tea leaves. By then I wasn't surprised at anything Ivy could do. Miss May got round to the fortune telling as she got round to most things, by first asking a favour.

'Darling matron,' she breathed, clutching my hand. 'I wonder if it would be asking too much of you to go into the town and bring me a small pot of fish paste and two iced buns?'

I had already been into town and brought her a sliver of steak for her lunch. It was never the bulk of the purchases that made shopping for Miss May a wearisome task, it was the time taken to execute the order that irked me sometimes, especially if the list she gave me was long. Her plaice had to be bought from the stall in the arcade, for no other reason than that the stall had once belonged to Miss May's mother's sister's son. The sliver of steak could only be guaranteed to melt in the mouth if it came from the butcher on the other side of the town from the arcade. The butcher was a distant relative of Miss May's cousin Sid who had met his end on a double-decker bus. Greengrocery only passed the freshness test if bought from the shop that had once been owned by Miss May's Great-Aunt Florence. The shop had changed hands many times since Florence started the business in a very small way by growing the produce in her kitchen garden and selling it to her neighbours at a copper or two above cost. But Miss May stayed loyal to family tradition. Not a potato would pass her lips unless she was sure it had come from Great-Aunt Florence's shop. Buying fish, meat and greengrocery for the gentle Miss May entailed a circular tour round the town.

When the first of the new supermarkets sprang up in the brand new precinct I spent a great deal of time telling Miss May that there was no longer any need to go to different shops for different things. But the thought of fish, meat and bananas being jumbled together on a shelf so confused her that I dropped the subject and gave her a cup of Milo to soothe her jangled nerves. There were aspects of modern living that Miss May would never understand. Decimal currency and supermarkets were amongst them.

'Are you expecting a visitor for tea?' I asked her, after I had promised faithfully that I would buy the buns at the bakery way beyond the butcher's shop, where everything was made on the premises and sliced bread might never have been invented.

'Mrs Koloski's coming,' she said, 'or Ivy, as she has asked me to call her. You remember I told you that we used to meet in the ambulance when she was going to the hospital with her legs? She called in yesterday and did a few little jobs which the home help hadn't time to do and we had a nice little chat about my troubles. It seems that she reads the tea leaves and she's promised to see if she can find out anything about an old friend of mine who emigrated to America a year or two ago. I haven't had a line from her since she went and I've been so worried about her. It would take a weight off my mind if Ivy could see her in the tea leaves and find out how she's getting on.'

'Does Ivy know her?' I asked, thinking that if she did it might make the tea-leaf reading easier. I sometimes had a nasty suspicious mind.

'She doesn't exactly know her,' replied Miss May. 'But I've told her so much about her that she couldn't fail to recognize her if she saw her at the bottom of the cup.' Despite what the tea leaves might tell her, Ivy appeared to require plenty of background history of her subject before she launched a full-scale search among the dregs.

The search produced excellent results. Ivy was able to see Miss May's friend quite clearly in the cup. She was radiant with health and happiness. Ivy could also see a Yorkshire terrier, two tabby cats and a canary. She said they were the spitting image of the dog, cats and canary which had had to be left behind when their mistress emigrated. Miss May had been so overcome when she described them to Ivy that she had to have a sniff of smelling salts to revive her.

She was delighted at Ivy's assurance that not only was her friend fit and well, but her new pets had become so dear to her that they had quite taken the place of the old ones. Miss May had lain awake at night fearing that in a country as large as America there would be no room for pets, and she knew how empty her friend's life would have been without them. Ivy, she said, had done more to give her restful nights than all the doctor's pills; but she still took the pills, just in case.

Over the months Ivy improved on her powers of clairvoyance. When she went visiting she took with her a pack of cards, shuffled them, spread them in

symbolic rows across the table and proceeded to fore-
tell the future. Her predictions were amazingly
accurate and almost always weighted on the side of
good fortune. When she told Mrs Smith that she
would shortly be getting a letter concerning a windfall,
Mrs Smith was inclined to scoff. She hadn't had a
letter for years except those threatening terrible things
unless she paid her bills. She made Ivy shuffle the cards
again but the result was the same. The king of hearts,
which Ivy said meant that she would be getting the
letter, was on the top of the pack.

The letter arrived the very next day. It said that as
Mrs Smith had recently celebrated her eightieth
birthday she had become eligible for the twenty-five
pence age allowance on top of her old age pension.

'Well, would you believe that?' said Ivy. 'I would
never have guessed you were anywhere near eighty.'
Mrs Smith had gone round boasting to everybody
about being eighty for weeks before she was.

Ivy went from strength to strength.

'A few of us are having a little get-together tonight,'
Mrs Turgoose announced when I was doing the round
one morning.

'That's nice, where are you having it?' I asked,
thinking in terms of a small banquet at the Wimpy bar

in the precinct. I knew that in the past Mrs Turgoose's idea of a get-together had been a drop of gin and a knees-up at a nearby pub or in a friend's front room. But those days were over, gone with the dawn of a new era of sedateness at the Lodge.

'We're having it at Ivy's place,' she said. 'She's holding one of those things where you all sit round the table with your eyes shut and she goes into a sort of trance and talks to people who have passed over. If she's lucky and in touch with them they talk back to her.'

'Oh, a seance,' I said.

'Pardon?' said Mrs Turgoose.

'It's called a seance,' I said. 'I've never been to one myself but I wouldn't mind coming if nobody objects. I didn't know Ivy was a medium, it's a wonder she hasn't mentioned it to me.'

'I don't know about her being one of them,' said Mrs Turgoose. 'All I know is that she says that if we tell her one or two things about our loved ones who have passed over she can arrange for us to have a word with them, or she'll have a word with them for us.'

'And who do you want to have a word with?' I asked.

'I haven't made up my mind yet,' she said. 'But I'm thinking of asking Ivy if she can find out what happened to the pair of gloves I lent Mrs Marsh not long before she died. I haven't set eyes on them since

245

the day I lent them to her. And there's the fur coat which my sister Ada said I could have if she went first. I never got it and I should like her word in front of witnesses that it's mine by rights. I've seen one of her daughters in it and I want to get the matter settled once and for all.'

I went to the seance and so did Mrs Turgoose, Miss Cromwell, Mrs James and, surprisingly, Mrs Dean. Miss Macintosh was in bed with a cold and Mrs Peters had cried off at the last minute saying that as there wasn't anybody in particular that she wanted to get in touch with she might as well stop at home and watch the telly.

Ivy started by giving us a cup of tea and a biscuit. Then she made us all huddle together round a small table with our eyes shut. She turned off the lights and I hitched a bit closer to Miss Cromwell. I could smell the moth balls on her clothes.

For a moment Ivy sat without saying anything. Then she took a deep breath and started to speak.

'Is there anybody sitting round this table who's lost somebody?' she asked, using her own voice as if it wasn't a seance but simply a few ladies huddled round a table. Nobody spoke but I felt Mrs Dean give a slight start. She was sitting on the other side of me from Miss Cromwell.

'If there is,' went on Ivy, 'I've been instructed to tell them that those they've lost are as right as rain and wish that those sitting round this table would stop dwelling on the past and blaming themselves for something that wasn't anybody's fault. What is to be will be and nothing can change it.'

She was quiet for a moment, then she drew in another deep breath. 'I'm getting a dog,' she said. This time it was Mrs James who gave a start. I'd got used to the darkness by now and saw her lean across the table as if she was trying to see what Ivy was looking at.

'It's an old dog,' said Ivy. 'But it looks very peaceful. I shouldn't be surprised if its time had come even before it was put down.' She paused again. 'Hang on,' she said sharply. 'There's a man with it. He's got it on a lead. Neither of them looks miserable to me.' Mrs James relaxed in her chair, then dabbed her eyes with her handkerchief.

But the seance wasn't over. 'There's a pair of gloves and an old fur coat floating in front of me,' said Ivy. 'The gloves are full of holes and the coat looks as if it's ready for the dustbin. I'm getting the lady who used to own the coat. She says I've to tell her sister, whoever that might be, that she's looking forward to seeing her soon.'

Ivy got up, turned on the lights and we all went home.

'I could have done without my sister Ada saying she'd see me soon,' said Mrs Turgoose the next day. 'She was always one to put her spoke in when it wasn't called for. Mind you, I was pleased about the coat. I can't wait to tell my niece that I know it's only fit for the dustbin. She's been going round in it as if she'd just bought it from 'arrods.'

'I've never believed in things like that before,' said Mrs Dean. 'But I could feel my daughter in the room last night. It was as if she was standing behind me telling me to stop blaming myself for her death.'

'And so you must,' I said. 'Nobody was to blame. Your son-in-law had a heart attack while he was driving the car and couldn't have done anything to save himself or your daughter.'

After she had stopped crying she told me the whole story. Deep down she had wanted to blame her son-in-law but she knew that her daughter had loved him. Somebody had to be blamed so she carried the burden herself.

The next time she visited the cemetery she took two bunches of flowers, one for her daughter and one for her son-in-law, and went on doing so until she could no longer get to their graves.

'Did you hear Ivy talking about that dog?' asked Mrs James. 'It was our old dog. I had her put down after my husband died because she went off for a week just before he died and he nearly went out of his mind. I never forgave her for it. I've often thought about it since. He wouldn't have liked me having her put down.'

'Never mind,' I said. 'According to Ivy they're both all right so I shouldn't think about it any more.'

The next day when I went to see her I noticed several framed photographs of the dog, her husband with the dog, and of her and her husband with the dog. They must have been hidden until then so that she wouldn't be reminded that she'd had the poor old thing put down. But from what I could see of it in the photographs Ivy had been right. If Lassie hadn't been put down she would most certainly have died of natural causes within a very short time.

'You don't really read the tea leaves and take messages from people who aren't there, do you?' I asked Ivy when we were having a cup of tea in her flat soon after the seance.

She didn't answer but took my cup from me and stared into the dregs. 'You'll be going on a journey soon,' she said, screwing up her eyes in an effort to concentrate on my future. 'I can see a lot of water and what looks like a boat.' There wasn't a soul at the Lodge who didn't know that at the end of the week I was off to the Isle of Wight for my annual holiday. I was about to tell Ivy what a phoney I thought she was when I thought of Mrs Dean. Phoney or not, Ivy had managed to find a way to bring her comfort, and Mrs James was a lot happier now that she knew her dog was happy and reunited with its master.

Ivy bent lower over my teacup, then looked at me.

'What's the matter?' I asked, forgetting for a moment that I knew she was a phoney and made it all up as she went along, helped considerably by the long chats she had with her neighbours, either as they sat on a bench in the porch, or while she did little odd jobs for them.

'There's something in here that I don't like the look of,' she said, gazing back at the tea leaves. 'It's a bit muzzy but it's there all right.'

'What is?' I asked, interested in spite of myself. 'Is the ferry boat going to capsize when we're halfway to Ryde?'

Ivy frowned at me for being flippant and upsetting her concentration. 'It's nothing to joke about,' she said. 'I can see you in bed with wires all round you.'

'You've been watching too much telly,' I told her. (She was an avid viewer of hospital dramas.) 'Or you're getting me mixed up with Mrs Smith.' Mrs Smith had slipped in her kitchen the week before, and was in hospital with her leg in traction.

'It's all right for you to snigger but things goes in threes. If you remember, there was Mrs Hankin last month who landed herself in hospital after she'd eaten a bit of chicken that wasn't cooked through. Then there was Mrs Smith and her leg last week and from what I can see in your tea leaves it could be your turn next.'

I laughed scornfully and went on my way. I might not have been so scornful if I'd known that Ivy's look into the tea leaves had given her a true picture of my future. But I didn't believe in fortune telling.

Chapter Thirteen

However close to the truth Ivy had come with her forecasting in my case, she had quite definitely got her facts wrong on something else. Mrs Hankin was not in hospital because she had eaten a piece of chicken that hadn't been cooked properly, she was there because the pains in her stomach, which she had been having since long before she ate the chicken, had suddenly got worse and an ambulance had to be sent for in the middle of one very wintry night.

After the doctors, whom she had stubbornly refused to see until it was too late, had finished diagnosing the pains, they told her that though they didn't think there was much for her to worry about they were going to keep her under observation for a while.

They didn't tell her that the pains would never go away, and she would need drugs in ever-increasing doses as the weeks that were left to her went by. Not all patients beg to be told the truth and bear up bravely when they hear that their days are numbered. Some prefer to go on thinking that they will be well again by next week, in a month or two or at the worst by this time next year. The doctors in their wisdom had decided that Mrs Hankin wouldn't benefit from being told that her illness was terminal.

She was a tall, thin woman, hair drawn back severely, her face heavily lined with the cares of a long life. She wasn't much interested in the things that were happening around her, preferring to dwell on things that had saddened her in the past, or, more rarely, on the few occasions when she had found happiness.

The two wars she had lived through had both brought her misery. Her father was killed in the first one, her brother and two sisters in the second. All the emotions of her drab life seemed to have been centred on the brother who was out walking his dog when the bomb fell. It was a very large bomb, big enough to kill not only him but his sisters and a great many others besides. Mrs Hankin was somewhere else when it happened but she always talked as if she would rather have been there. Mrs Hankin lived with her mother until death took her as well.

She had worked in a munitions factory while the war was on, and when the war ended and the factory started manufacturing pots and pans instead of shells she stayed there, bossing the bosses while she polished their offices and made them cups of tea. When they pensioned her off, strings were pulled and she came to live at the Lodge. She arrived there with nothing much to show for a life spent in doing her duty to others.

She was a religious woman, fearing God whom she knew as a grim-faced Father, crushing the world under his thumb and relentlessly punishing wrong-doers. Disease and pestilence were sent to scourge the unrighteous, even if the righteous got embroiled as well. Children starved in distant lands for some inscrutable, divine purpose.

When I asked her why the Lord, who was reputed to have known about the fall of a single sparrow, seemed to turn a blind eye while the children died through no fault of their own, Mrs Hankin had a ready answer. She told me that she well remembered her father beating her and her brother and sisters for the most trifling offence and sending them to bed hungry, sometimes for sins they hadn't even committed. But it hadn't occurred to them to question his love. They had bent over meekly under the chastisement and gone to bed hungry, knowing that he, being their father, knew best. God, she said, meted out punishment in the very same way, though on a grander scale, of course.

I still thought that sending children to bed without any supper was a somewhat grim way of showing affection.

Mrs Hankin never sat on the verandah with Ivy and the others. Even Ivy couldn't get through to her when she went up and offered her friendship. She was civil to her neighbours but exchanged no more than a word or two when she met them while she was on her way to the shops, or shared a washing line with them on Mondays. She cooked her small meals, swept and polished her flat, and spent most of her days looking into the past with pain-filled eyes. The pain was in her mind until it became the pain of her terminal illness.

There were those at the Lodge who vaguely remembered seeing Mrs Hankin pushing her mother round the town in a wheelchair; her mother was an invalid for many years before she died. But even Mrs Turgoose, who could usually be relied upon to give me a case history of every resident, had nothing much to say on the subject of Mrs Hankin. The things she told me were things I had heard already from others round the Lodge, and from Mrs Hankin herself.

'I remember the night the bomb fell and all those people, including her brother and two sisters, got killed. It was a terrible night, that was. There was a family that had only just come down from London to get away from the bombs and every one of them got killed. I don't remember seeing Mrs Hankin about much after that until she started pushing her mother up the High Street in a wheelchair. She came to the Darby and Joan club once, I remember, but she wasn't the sort to join in things so she never came again. You have to join in with the others if you belong to a club. It's like everything else in this life, you only get out of it what you put in. It's not a bit of use sitting there waiting for others to make the first move.'

I enjoyed listening to Mrs Hankin talking about the happier times in her life. Her father's name was Barnabas, and though his family wasn't Jewish they all had Jewish names. There was her Aunt Leah, Uncle Benjie, and her cousins Levi, Isaiah and Joseph. There had been a Ruth and a Rachel as well, but they died of diphtheria while still in their cradles.

They had lived in the pit-scarred outskirts of Nottingham and Mrs Hankin remembered the long exciting train journey from where she lived near London to the far-removed world of her biblically named relations.

The men worked down the pit and came home black and hungry. Every day Aunt Leah had made five large Yorkshire puddings and five creamy rice puddings, one for each of the breadwinners. She spent her life scrubbing their coal-black backs in a tin bath in front of the kitchen fire, scrubbing their coal-black clothes, and cooking mounds of food to feed them. Having five miners in the family left little time for hobbies. Mrs Hankin said it would have been nice if Ruth and Rachel had lived. They would have been a great help to their mother when they got old enough to share in the washing and cooking.

The day her uncle Benjamin died she was in chapel with her aunt. She said she could still hear the women crying and the men swearing after somebody rushed in to say there had been an explosion down the pit. Uncle Benjamin was one of the first to be brought up.

After a suitable period of mourning Leah married Chas. He had been Ben's best friend and the marriage had been arranged long before the accident happened. Leah could have taken her pick of either of them from the time she reached marriageable age but she had chosen Ben. It was an understood thing between them that Chas should stay single to be by her side if Ben was taken first. When he went home to Leah, black and hungry, it could still have been Ben sitting in the bath having his back scrubbed.

Mrs Hankin told me more stories about her childhood when I went to see her in hospital. On her mother's side there had been a cousin called Jane. Her young man had promised undying love, before going off to be a soldier, but he got a girl in trouble almost as soon as he put on his uniform, and married her. Jane ran away from home. She was found wandering in a town close by, looking for her lost love. When they eventually persuaded her to come home she gathered together everything that was hers in the house, took it to a large upstairs room and shut herself away, only emerging when she could be absolutely sure that there was nobody in the house but her, or maybe just her mother.

I was taken back to my own childhood when Mrs Hankin told me how every summer, her father, mother and brother, each riding a bicycle with her and her sisters strapped on carriers at the back, had sped along lanes lined with sweet-smelling hedgerows on the way to the rambling farmhouse where their cousin Jane lived. As well as having a child clinging on behind, Mr Hankin balanced a wicker basket containing their clothes on the front of his bike.

As a child, I had been taken on holiday in similar fashion, riding behind my father's bicycle while my mother had the wicker basket strapped to hers. We had skimmed uphill and downhill through Lincolnshire lanes, past apple-scented orchards and across flat fenland, I and the wicker basket bumping and shifting as my parents pedalled over ruts and dried-out puddle holes.

As Mrs Hankin and her family got nearer to the farmhouse the children excitedly speculated on whether they would get a fleeting glimpse of cousin Jane that year. But it was only on the rarest occasions that they saw her at the window of the room upstairs, magically mysterious to them, brought there in spite of herself by the sound of their voices as they played round the pump near the kitchen door. There were hens in the yard where the pump was, said Mrs Hankin, Rhode Island Reds, White Wyandottes and dear little bantams. There were geese as well, great, dangerous screeching things that sent the children running into the house in fear. The hens also ran into the house, and pecked round the floor in search of crumbs dropped from a previous meal. This aunt, said Mrs Hankin, hadn't been houseproud. She let the hens stay where they were until they got too daring and fluttered onto the table in search of bigger crumbs. Then she feebly flapped at them with a tea towel, sending them back into the yard until they thought it was safe to come in for another feed.

'What happened to cousin Jane in the end?' I asked Mrs Hankin, rousing her from a memory that had softened her face into a gentle smile.

'Now that was a very funny thing,' she said, nodding her head reflectively. 'Nobody would ever have dreamed she would have turned out the way she did after all those years of shutting herself away in that big room upstairs. She was still there when her father died, and after all but one of her brothers were married.'

When her mother died Jane came downstairs, took over the house and helped her bachelor brother to run the farm. It was almost as if she had never shut herself away. But she never bought herself anything new. She tended the cows and helped with the harvest in the same clothes she had been wearing when she ran away from home. Though out of date, they still fitted her perfectly.

She didn't speak to anybody unless it was strictly necessary but she kept the house sparkling clean and never allowed the hens across the back doorstep. Her brother had to go outside if he wanted to smoke his pipe.

Only once did she go back to her old way of living and that was when the man who had jilted her came to the village to look up some of his relations. He had been in India for many years. He and Jane met by chance in the place where he used to take her when he was making his false promises and she turned straight round and went back to the room at the top of the house. She didn't stay there long, though; she knew her brother needed her.

The man hadn't even recognized her. When somebody told him who she was and how she had behaved after he went to be a soldier, he could hardly believe his ears. He said he'd never intended the little flirtation he'd had with her to go any further. And as for marrying her, why, such a thing had never crossed his mind. He never would have thought she'd taken a harmless bit of fun so seriously. He was thunderstruck, he said. He didn't come back to the village again.

I let Mrs Hankin finish telling me the story of her cousin Jane. Then I asked her if there was a lavatory with three holes down the yard at the farmhouse. After a moment she said that now she came to think of it, there was.

'But how did you know about that?' she asked. I told her that I also used to have an aunt who lived in a rambling farmhouse where there was an outside lavatory with three holes, graded small, medium and large. Then we talked about life as it was when every country homestead had hams and sides of bacon hanging like old masters on the living room walls, to be cut into when a sizzling breakfast or a substantial high tea was required. I grew up in a rather aging house where once a year our kitchen had been full of the smell of the good things my mother made after the pig, which my father had fattened in a sty close to the kitchen door, was killed for Christmas. I went back in time with Mrs Hankin and topped each of her nostalgic memories with another of my own.

It was while she was stubbornly refusing to see a doctor about the pain she was getting that a man came to my door, established that I was the matron, and asked me if there was a woman called Mrs Hankin living in the Lodge. As there seemed to be nothing sinister about him I showed him where she lived. The next day she seemed puzzled.

'You know that man you sent over yesterday, well, I still don't know what he came for.'

I looked at her in alarm, wondering if I'd done the right thing in sending him across.

'He said something about being sent by the Prudential to see if I wanted to take out another policy. But I told him I wasn't interested. I've paid twopence a week since Mother died, which will cover the cost when I go. Then he asked me if he could come again sometime, just to have a chat. I got sharp with him then and sent him about his business. He said he was sorry he'd troubled me and hoped I hadn't minded him coming. It's a funny thing, you know, but when I was thinking about it afterwards it struck me that he wasn't an insurance man at all. He didn't have the proper papers. But he was a decent sort of man and I suppose I could have been a bit nicer to him than I was.'

I told her not to worry about him; if it had been important he'd have stated his business more straightforwardly. It was I who worried, wondering what the purpose of his visit had been and whether he would come back again. As matron of the Lodge it was my duty to protect the residents from unwanted callers.

By the following day Mrs Hankin had solved the problem of the insurance man. When I went to see her she was sitting at her table surrounded by photographs. She looked as if she'd been crying for a long time.

'It was my son,' she said the moment I walked in.

I sank into the chair I always sat in when it seemed I would spend longer with Mrs Hankin than the time I normally allowed for a routine visit.

'I don't understand,' I said. 'Who was your son?'

I wondered whether she had suddenly started hearing voices or imagining things. Mrs Hunt had heard voices and used to have terrible rows with them. I had worked with the elderly long enough to know that hearing voices wasn't necessarily a symptom of mental derangement or advanced senility. Neither did I send for a psychiatrist the moment I heard a resident having a little chat with herself. I often said a few words to myself when under stress, and I was far from being senile.

'That man who said he'd come about the insurance was my son,' said Mrs Hankin. She said it in such a sad and hopeless way that I put out my hand and laid it on hers. She picked up one of the photographs and stared at it with tear-filled eyes.

'But you haven't got a son,' I said, 'so why do you say a thing like that?'

She handed me the photograph. It was of a wedding group. I recognized the bride at once. She pointed to the groom.

'That was my husband,' she said, unnecessarily. 'We hadn't been married more than a few months when I found out he was already married. I shall never forget the day his wife turned up with their two children. Somebody had sent her a cutting out of the paper about our wedding. They had parted after the last child was born but they were still legally married. He went back to her and I never saw him again. He was up for bigamy, of course, but he behaved like a gentleman in the end and I didn't have to go to court. But I had a son within the year. Mother had him put into a children's home. I didn't want her to but things were different then and I couldn't have afforded to keep him. That was him that came here yesterday.'

'But how can you be so sure?' I said. 'He was in his fifties and you say yourself that you didn't see your son after he was sent to the home. You couldn't possibly have known him after all these years.'

'I'm sure,' she said. 'As sure as I am that I'm sitting here. I kept wondering yesterday who he reminded me of. This morning it came to me. He's the double of his father. If only it could have come to me sooner. He'll have gone away thinking I've rejected him again as I rejected him after he was born.' She put her head down on the table and wept.

When the storm was over we looked at the photograph together and I had to admit that there was something about the groom's bearing and his thick-set frame that bore a likeness to the man who came to ask where Mrs Hankin lived.

'Even the things I said to him might have made him think that I knew who he was but didn't want to own him. I told him I wasn't interested in what he had to say and that I didn't want to be bothered with him coming back. I remember the way he said he was sorry to have troubled me and he hoped I hadn't minded him calling.' She was still weeping when I left her.

The thought of her twice-rejected son haunted Mrs Hankin. She went over and over with me the story of his infancy and her heartbreak at having to part with her baby son. She went from that to the day he came to see her and she sent him away. She couldn't forgive herself for that. 'Surely there should have been something in me to tell me that he was my own flesh and blood,' she said wearily whenever I was with her. 'It's as if I'd had him adopted because I didn't want him, then turned him away because I refused to admit he was mine. I wonder if he'll ever come back again.'

Mrs Hankin was in hospital when her son came back again. Miss Macintosh saw him knocking at the door of her empty flat and sent him across to me. The hospital had just rung me to say that her condition was rapidly deteriorating and by the time we got to her bedside she knew neither of us.

'I shall always regret that I didn't make myself known to her the first time I came,' he said as he drove me back to the Lodge after we had sat and watched her die. 'I foolishly thought that she might have had some idea who I was but she believed me when I told her I was an insurance agent. I was no more than a stranger to her.'

I waited until we got back to the Lodge before I told him otherwise. Such a piece of information required more concentration than he could give it while driving a car through the rush-hour traffic.

'You weren't a stranger to her,' I told him. 'She knew almost as soon as you'd gone that you were her son. She grieved ever since that her instinct hadn't told her sooner. She never stopped reproaching herself for sending you away. She thought you'd think she knew and had deliberately turned her back on you.'

I gave him the photographs that had proved to Mrs Hankin who he was and he told me how he always intended trying to find her but first one thing had cropped up, then another, until finally it was too late. He was as upset at not coming sooner as Mrs Hankin had been at not knowing him when he was there.

He came to his mother's funeral, and brought with him his son and daughter and two grandchildren. I was sorry that she couldn't have known. It would have made up for a lot of things she had missed in life.

Part Four

Part Four

Chapter Fourteen

WHEN MRS TURGOOSE was nearing her ninetieth birthday Ivy Koloski and one or two others round the Lodge approached me with the suggestion that we should have a party to celebrate the occasion. They had already talked about it among themselves and had made provisional plans, including wild schemes such as throwing open the Lodge to all and sundry, holding a fancy-dress ball and, more down to earth, a simple tea party on the verandah with Mrs Turgoose as the honoured guest.

I gave the matter some thought before finally agreeing to the tea party. Such a thing had never been done before, partly because those who had birthdays were usually made much of by friends and relatives, who arrived at the Lodge with bedsocks and tins of mint humbugs, and partly because there had been no Ivy to organize the event. Mrs Turgoose had nobody closer to her than the niece who got in first and claimed the moth-eaten fur coat which Ivy had seen at the seance. The niece wasn't likely to turn up at the Lodge with bedsocks and humbugs or a cake with nine candles, one for every ten years of Mrs Turgoose's action-packed life: at least those who believed the tales she told them might have thought that hardly a day had gone by without something spectacular happening to Mrs Turgoose.

I believed the tales myself until she held me spell-bound with an unbelievable story of how she had been to a garden party given by one of the highest in the land, if not the highest. After much probing from me and some reluctant retracting from her it was finally established that she had gone with the Sunshine Club to visit the gardens of some very minor royalties, the proceeds of their hospitality being donated to the District Nurses' Association. Without the probing I would have been left with a clear picture of Mrs Turgoose, in a large floppy hat and trailing dress, curt-seying to Her Majesty at a Buckingham Palace garden party. It wasn't that she deliberately set out to deceive, but she had the gift of the gab and could turn the most mundane happening into breathtaking drama.

After I had conferred with the administrative committee and gone into one or two details with Ivy I gave the party the go-ahead. The details I went into with Ivy were the same as those which the committee had gone into with me. It was to be understood by all the party-goers that there should be no unseemly revelling on the verandah, nothing stronger than lemonade to be served and everything to be cleared up when the party was over so that Stew wouldn't give in his notice, complaining of being overworked. I promised the committee, and Ivy promised me, that the rules would be adhered to.

The birthday celebration was to be a big surprise, not a word of it to reach Mrs Turgoose's ears until the time came for her to be led to the feast. Those able and willing were to make whatever contribution they could in the way of comestibles, shop bought or home baked. As Mrs Turgoose's birthday was early in June the porch doors were to be propped open and a buffet meal laid on the table where Stew kept his pot plants. If he did his job properly the verandah would be bright with baskets of scarlet geraniums and trailing lobelia.

Stew had taken over the gardener's job as well as his own until we got a new man. He knew less about gardening than he knew about space travel and it wasn't long before the shrubs and plants which the old gardener had tended with such knowledgeable pride showed signs of curling up and dying under his heavy hand. The grass went yellow and the roses were thick with greenfly. But Stew kept on trying. By the time the new man arrived everything had stopped growing.

There was some guarded excitement among the residents at the prospect of a celebration, the like of which had never been known before at the Lodge. Spurred on by Ivy they committed themselves to donating fairy cakes, jellies and jam tarts, and a bit of sugar or a drop of milk. Ivy was going to supply the tea.

Even Mrs Peters showed some interest. I was uncharitable enough to think that there might be an underlying reason for this. She was a year or two off ninety but not too far off to start paving the way for a similar party when her day dawned. Though she had sons and daughters to enjoy the pleasure of her company at birthdays and other celebratory occasions, their pleasure was often marred by a habit she had of stirring up strife when the merrymaking was at its height. They would be only too happy to have the responsibility of trying to please her taken off their shoulders. And she would find just as much to carp about no matter whose table her feet were under. Ivy had done a lot to sweeten her temper but she still had a long way to go.

'It's no use coming to me for anything,' she said when I was touting for volunteers to make dainties. 'I wouldn't lift a finger for Polly Turgoose. It's not that

I've anything against her but she's a backbiting, scandal-mongering woman who's caused more trouble down at the club than all the others rolled into one. I daresay there'll be those that can't stand the sight of her who'll be only too ready to push themselves forward on her birthday, if only to get a bit of jelly and custard. Well, I shan't be one of them. I shall be at the party of course, if only to see her make a fool of herself as she did at the last Masonic Christmas dinner.' I winced at the memory.

The annual dinner laid on by the Masons had, until the previous Christmas, gone off without a hitch: or without a hitch big enough to cause questions to be asked by the charitable body. But Mrs Turgoose got carried away the previous Christmas and brought disgrace to us all. As well as the glass of sherry we were given after we had relinquished our coats, she had foolishly allowed the waitress at her table to fill up her wine glass more than once. It had gone to her head and even before the pudding was served she stood up and insisted that we should all join hands and sing Auld Lang Syne.

Mrs Peters and others looked on with various degrees of coldness while a few of us sang and got into a terrible muddle about which arm should be crossed over which. Miss May had come over queer and had to be given brandy, and Mrs Dean was so unutterably shocked by Mrs Turgoose's inebriated behaviour that she demanded to be taken home before the Masonic presents were given out. It was a most unfortunate evening and I got a stern letter from the committee rebuking me for allowing things to get out of hand.

I passed on the rebuke to Mrs Turgoose and told her that unless she promised to behave herself there would be no question of her ever going to the Masonic dinner again. She said she wouldn't promise no such thing, and what could she do if the waitress kept topping up her glass when she wasn't looking? I made a note to remind the waitresses at the next dinner that it was strictly one glass per resident: any leftovers to be discreetly shared between them and me.

I was still thinking about Mrs Turgoose's fall from grace when Mrs Peters remembered Ivy's kindness to her. She reached up to a shelf in her dresser and took down a very large teapot.

'I don't mind you borrowing this for Polly Turgoose's do,' she said, dusting the lid and handing me the pot. It's got no spout but so long as you remember to hold something under when you pour it should be all right.'

I thanked her for her generous offer and said words to the effect that we wouldn't have known which way to turn without it. I didn't tell her that it was the fourth teapot we'd got on loan, with the prospect of several more before the big day arrived. I knew how vital it was to say nothing that could cause bad feeling before the festivities commenced, however much they might degenerate over the tea table. In a final burst of philanthropy Mrs Peters offered us the set of fruit dishes which she said she never used as most of them were chipped. I refused the dishes on the pretext that they were much too grand to be put at risk in the hurly-burly of a verandah party. I knew that even one more chip, added to the many I could see, would have to be accounted for when the dishes were returned.

The preparations for the party were going well when Mrs Turgoose started to smell a rat. 'What's going on round here?' she asked me on the day before her birthday. She sat huddled in front of her fire wrapped in as many shawls as Miss May wore in the early days of summer. There were greeting cards on the mantelpiece and fresh bunches of plastic flowers on the dresser. They contrasted sharply with the tired-looking, older displays.

'There's nothing going on round here,' I said, thankful to be able to tell the truth; all the volunteers had gone home for their tea. She gave me a suspicious look and sniffed loudly.

'There's something going on that I don't understand. I may be old but I'm not daft. There hasn't been so many folks stampeding up and down this verandah since the Coronation, when we all flocked into Kate Saywell's place to watch it on her set. She was the only one round here that had a set and we were packed like sardines. As I remember she passed away soon after. And not a bit of wonder. It was enough to kill anybody sitting from eleven in the morning or sooner to when they'd all stopped coming out on that balcony of theirs. I don't mind telling you that I had to have the doctor in about my waterworks. They were never the same after being bottled up like they was for nearly a day. Nobody could go in case we missed something while we was going.

'I reckon Ivy Koloski's at the bottom of whatever's going on round here,' she continued. 'She must be holding a lot of them seance things of hers, there's first one and then another sneaking in and out of her place. I notice I don't get an invite. Well, she knows what she can do. I was never one to push my nose in where it wasn't wanted.'

Ivy was the self-appointed organizer of the forthcoming event. She had hand-picked her committee, drawing on ladies who had some special skill like being able to fold paper napkins, or were willing to run when she cracked the whip. She cracked the whip a lot in the time leading up to the party, revealing a strength of mind which she had cultivated through years of dealing with argumentative men at the betting shop.

Because of her long office experience Miss Macintosh was unanimously elected as secretary and treasurer combined. It was her job to do the paper-work, which included lists of things that were borrowed to ensure that everything would be returned to its rightful owner, and to collect money from people like Miss May who contributed sixpence towards bread for the sandwiches and sixpence towards fish paste. Miss Macintosh was also responsible for getting names of those willing to cut the bread, butter it and spread the fish paste. Making it three separate tasks insured against anybody complaining that they were doing the donkey work. In her capacity as treasurer Miss Macintosh raffled a tablet of soap I had given her the Christmas before. The raffle brought in tenpence and I won the soap.

Being in better shape physically than the other members of the committee, Miss Cromwell was dele-gated to helping Stew carry chairs onto the verandah to supplement the wooden benches. Mrs James was put in charge of the flower vase. Stew's plants still hadn't got over the shock of having an amateur inter-fering with their established way of life and the hanging baskets had failed to come up to expectations. There were so few roses that Stew counted them every day and would have noticed at once if one had been appropriated.

Mrs Peters wasn't asked to do anything and neither did she volunteer her services. She sat in at all the committee meetings giving advice that wasn't taken and throwing cold water on ideas put forward by others.

Another who regularly attended the meetings but wasn't asked to do anything was Mrs Dean. Her habit of mislaying things had worsened over the years. It was a foregone conclusion that nothing she was put in charge of would get done; she would either forget it entirely or lose something vital to the smooth running of the party. She caused a terrible rumpus when the steering committee was being formed by suddenly discovering that the ring she wore on her little finger was no longer there. The meeting was held up while a search was made. The floor was gone over inch by inch. The settee where Mrs Dean had been sitting had its loose covers torn off, hands were thrust down amongst the fluff, bringing up a considerable sum in old money, a very old button hook, a quantity of knit-ting needles, an empty wallet, but no ring.

After the floor had been gone over again everybody trooped out of Ivy's place and retraced Mrs Dean's journey from her flat to Ivy's several times. They lifted up stones, forked over the debris in the gully and even ran their hands along the top of the windows on the verandah in case by some miracle the ring had bounced when it fell and come to rest up there.

Mrs Dean found her ring in the velvet-lined ring box where she always kept it when she hadn't got it on. Luckily she made the discovery before she had time to post the angry letters she had written to the charitable body, Scotland Yard and Her Majesty the Queen.

In the light of all this Ivy wisely decided to delete Mrs Dean's name from the list of volunteers for the steering committee.

It wasn't to be expected that Miss May would be able to take an active part in the frenzied preparations. She was sadly aware of her inadequacies and fervently expressed the wish that she should be 'taken' before she became even more of a burden to me and everybody else. After she had dabbed her eyes and blown her nose she went with faltering feet to a drawer. From it she brought several crocheted doilies and a very large tablecloth edged with lace of an intricate pattern, depicting the flags of the nations. Miss May told me, weeping again, that she had crocheted the lace to commemorate the armistice in 1918. It was over-blued with countless washings in the family laundry but perfectly preserved.

On the morning of her birthday Mrs Turgoose fell off a chair and broke her wrist. She had clambered on the chair to get a better look at Stew who was hanging a Chinese lantern in the porch. I went with her to the hospital and stayed there while they put a plaster on her arm and made sure she was well enough to be sent home.

The party was over when we got back and except for the Chinese lantern the porch showed no sign that anything unusual had taken place. Ivy took me aside and whispered that everything had gone off well and a perfectly splendid time had been had by all, except Mrs Peters who complained about the sandwiches saying that she had never cared for bloater paste and them that got all the salmon ones must have known what they were doing and sat at the end of the table where the salmon ones were.

Ivy had saved a few sandwiches, a bit of fruit cake and a small basin of jelly and custard, but Mrs Turgoose went straight to bed and I ate her share as well as my own. She never knew about the party that had been given in her honour. To have told her would only have added insult to injury, and with the excitement of breaking her wrist she had quite forgotten what day it was.

Chapter Fifteen

THE SUCCESS OF the birthday celebrations went to Ivy's head. No sooner had Stew removed the solitary paper lantern from the porch than Ivy set her mind to organizing other events. Scarcely a week went by when she wasn't pinning notices in prominent places reminding the residents that their company was requested at some function or other. None of the things she organized were on the grand scale of her first ambitious enterprise but she rallied the residents round and encouraged them to participate in various activities which she had laid on for their benefit. She even tried to arrange a coach party to go to Epsom on Derby Day, but nobody appended her name to the piece of paper which Ivy passed round outlining her plans. She was obliged to cancel the thirty-two seater coach she had optimistically ordered to be on the forecourt at a specified time. The coach firm involved hadn't been able to make head or tail of her letters and had disregarded them, so nothing was lost.

When Ivy saw that nobody was interested in a day at the races she asked me whether I thought it would be all right if she and Miss Cromwell went on their own. I said that in view of the crush there always was on the Downs, and Ivy's bad legs which, though better than they were, still troubled her if she stood on them too long, I felt it would be better if they watched the race on television, pointing out that they would see more of it, even though all the jockeys would look alike in black and white. To make up for the disappointment I gave Ivy permission to organize a sweepstake, as I had done until the charitable body took exception to the matron doing anything so unmatronlike.

As well as running the sweepstake Ivy surreptitiously took small bets for residents who were not above going to her door with folded slips of paper. When the horses they fancied failed to come up to their expectations Ivy generously refunded their money in full. When they did she confused the punters with a complicated explanation of two-way bets, accumulator bets and other ways of betting which left the winner with no winnings.

Rumour had it that she was occasionally seen sidling into the shop on the High Street that had belonged to her before it grew out of all recognition. Mrs Turgoose, who started the rumour, remarked cattily that she no doubt received preferential treatment from the present owners, her being in the trade so to speak and bookies having a reputation for favouring some and handing out large sums of money while turning others away without a penny. She had lost her faith in bookmakers after placing a shilling on a horse that came in an easy first at the winning post. Unfortunately he had arrived there riderless, but Mrs Turgoose maintained that since it was the horse she had put her money on and not the jockey she should have got some return for the shilling which now lined the bookmaker's pocket.

According to Mrs Turgoose, Miss Cromwell got preferential treatment as well. Mrs Turgoose's home help had seen her in the baker's shop on Grand National day, buying buns as if money grew on trees. I reprimanded the home help for discussing one resident with another and reminded her that Miss Cromwell was fond of buns and bought a bag of them most days. It was sheer coincidence that she had chosen that particular occasion to buy two sorts.

Despite the trickle of residents that wound its way to her door for different purposes, Ivy's greatest triumph lay in the intimate little get togethers she had in her own small flat. As the evenings drew in and it started to get too chilly for elderly ladies to sit outside after tea Ivy invited them in for a game of whist, a hand of dominoes, a beetle drive or some competitive board game such as ludo or draughts. Space being limited the invitations were issued in strict rotation and the guests sat, elbows well tucked in and knees pressed to knees, round the miniature refectory table in Ivy's dining area.

The responsibility for supplying the refreshments was supposed to be shared equally between the guests. This gave rise to a certain amount of friction amongst those who sat round the table. Miss Cromwell, being Mrs Koloski's best friend because of the sporting interests they had in common, wasn't put on the roster. Though turning up at every function she never once brought anything to eat. Those who did found it most irritating to see her dipping into the biscuits, picking out her favourites and leaving the duller ones for them. They may have forgiven her, but they could never forget the tyrant she had been until Ivy arrived to give her other things to think of than storming along the verandah, slamming doors and upsetting everybody.

Miss Cromwell still had an occasional lapse when she donned her gaberdine coat and little round hat and strode out with her black bag, thinking that she was the matron. But she had lost her dominion over the residents and instead of shrinking back when she appeared on the scene and ringing their bells for me when she pushed past them, forcing them into the gully, they stood their ground and made some jocular remark which brought her back to reality. Somehow she didn't look as large then as she did when she was being a matron.

Miss Macintosh had been reluctant at first to accept Ivy's invitation to one of her soirees. She was of a shy retiring nature and not a good mixer unless she could relax, knowing that she didn't have to make scintillating conversation. But after Ivy had assured her that she needn't talk if she didn't want to and would only be expected to sit at the table and make up a foursome at ludo, she said she would be happy to attend when her name came up on the roster. She expressed her willingness to supply the refreshments when it was her turn.

Thereafter she went regularly, sometimes wearing the dress and jacket which she and I had examined for moth holes when she was worrying about what to wear for the first Christmas dinner given us by the Masons. The ensemble was all of twenty years old, but wearing it gave a sense of occasion to what otherwise might have been a rather ordinary game of ludo. Miss Macintosh confessed to me once that the outings to Ivy's place had become the high spots in her life, anticipated with pleasure and looked back on afterwards with a nice feeling of having been somewhere and done something. She enjoyed them even more after Ivy added lotto to her list of entertainments. Miss Macintosh said she knew it was the same as bingo but she didn't feel nearly as sinful playing it in Ivy's flat as she would have done at the bingo hall in the town. I occasionally dropped in for a game myself.

Mrs Peters had needed no persuading to take her place at the table. She saw it as the opportunity of a lifetime to have a battle of wits as well as words with her neighbours. She cheated so shamelessly at whichever game was being played that Ivy was petitioned by the other participants to strike her name off the roster. But Ivy was too kind-hearted to do a thing like that. She pretended not to hear when Mrs Peters shouted 'House' on a number that hadn't been called, and suggested they should all stop for a cup of tea when her huffing, revoking, and wrongfully sending her opponent's ludo back home threatened to disrupt the evening. Ivy had a wonderful way with people.

Every so often, in response to popular request, she held one of her seances. These had come a long way from the rather amateur show she put on when she was comforting Mrs Dean and easing Mrs Turgoose's anxiety about her late sister's fur coat. They had gone from strength to strength and were now darkly mysterious affairs that relied on much heavy breathing accompanied by hollow voices in a minor key to get their messages across. Not only were the voices in a minor key but they spoke in a strange tongue which only Ivy could understand. To the others sitting round the table it was an unintelligible jumble. But after long and pregnant pauses Ivy freely translated the utterances and passed the messages on to her audience.

As at the simpler seances, the messages owed their origins to the scraps of information that were bandied about on the bench in the porch, at the Senior Citizens' Club or during a shopping expedition in the town; but Ivy, faintly outlined under the dim light of a heavily shaded bulb, sporting a curiously shaped turban-like hat and a string of multi-coloured beads, created an aura that dispelled the doubts of all but the most sceptic that her information came from any other source than her spirit guide.

She only started to have a spirit guide after attendances at the less sophisticated seances had begun to drop off. He made his appearance very suddenly one evening, nearly frightening Mrs James, Mrs Dean and

Miss Macintosh to death. He had been summoned by Ivy to answer a tricky question that Mrs James had asked concerning the old gardener. She was anxious to know whether he was allowed to have an allotment in the place he went to after he died. She wouldn't have dreamed of asking, she said, but since Ivy had told her about the old dog and how happy it was it had occurred to her that she might be able to get in touch with the gardener.

Ivy leaned back in her chair, said several things in one of the strange languages and waited. Suddenly from somewhere in her direction came a deep sepulchral voice. It went on talking for a few minutes, after which Ivy sat forward and explained that it was her spirit guide who had spoken. He had told Ivy to tell Mrs James that he had been in touch with the old gardener, who assured him that he had unlimited scope for producing prize-winning blooms, the weather was always perfect and not a greenfly in sight.

Another question asked by Mrs James, after she had recovered from the shock of having the first one answered, brought the information, through the spirit guide, that her late husband knew all about her making steak and kidney pies for the old gardener; the two men had met and were now the best of friends. This cheered Mrs James immensely. She admitted to me afterwards that she had sometimes felt guilty at having another man's feet under her table. She was deeply grateful to Ivy's spirit guide for letting her know that her husband hadn't minded.

Neither Mrs Peters nor Mrs Turgoose believed a word about the visitor from beyond the grave. They had at the start but Ivy went overboard and ruined things for them.

'If you ask me anything it's all a load of eyewash,' said Mrs Turgoose after she heard at one of the seances that her husband was well and happy and had sent her his love. 'He was as miserable as sin and never happy unless he was moaning about something. He's hardly likely to have changed that much. And as for him sending me his love, you can take that with a pinch of salt. He was fonder of that old horse of his than he was of me. If he sent his love to anybody, which I strongly doubt, him not being given to using language like that, it would have been to his nag. The one that did the milk round with him to the day he died. And considering that it was on its last legs then it must be up there with him now, if they've managed to find each other among the crowds. I can just see them both sitting on a cloud playing their harps.' She nudged me and I smiled faintly.

Mrs Peters had tossed her head and stormed out of

a seance after Ivy told her that according to a message she was just getting there were big things afoot for Mrs Peters and she would shortly be going somewhere where hers would be one of the few white faces amongst a throng of darker skins. Mrs Peters had never set foot on foreign soil in her life and didn't intend to now, not at her time in life.

She didn't have to. Shortly after the seance her son plucked up courage to tell his mother he was moving to Birmingham. When he had got his house in order he fetched her to set her seal of disapproval on it. She came back stunned by the sights she had seen.

'That's the last time they'll get me there,' she said. 'The streets are swarming with people who look just like that young Indian doctor who came to see me when I was having a nervous breakdown.' She hadn't had a nervous breakdown, but she almost gave him one.

'How did you know her son was moving and where he was moving to?' I asked Ivy after she had finished reading my palm and warning me yet again that there was something she didn't like the look of. There was apparently a break in my health line which shouldn't have been there.

'I didn't know he was moving,' she said, sounding embarrassed. 'I knew no more about it than she did. It was him,' she said, 'the spirit guide. He told me. And I don't mind admitting to you that it gave me quite a turn when I heard him.'

'But I thought he was always telling you things,' I said with a touch of sarcasm. She didn't answer for a moment, then she took a deep breath and confessed all. The story was as wild as any that Mrs Turgoose had ever told me.

'It was me all the time,' she said. 'I just brought him in to liven things up and to make the seances seem more real. I went to one once years ago, and the woman there had a spirit guide. He was some sort of Red Indian with a funny name. I never said anything to hurt anybody. All I wanted was to tell them things that would make them happy. Mrs James was a lot happier after I told her about the old dog, and how her husband had got friendly with the gardener. And Mrs Dean might still have been going round with a long face if I hadn't told her I'd had a word with her daughter. And I told Miss May what she wanted to know about that friend of hers in America. You can't accuse me of doing anybody any harm.'

'So,' I said, 'what happened the night you told Mrs Peters about the place her son was going to?' Ivy gave me a troubled look.

'It wasn't me that night,' she said. 'I was just getting

ready to do my deep voice when this other voice started telling me that Mrs Peters's son was moving to Birmingham where all the immigrants were. I just passed on the message, but I wrapped it up a bit, knowing how funny she can be about foreigners.'

I began to feel rather alarmed. I wondered what the charitable body would say when I told them that one of the residents was psychic and had a spirit guide who brought her messages from another world.

'Why didn't any of the others hear the voice?' I asked her. I wanted to assemble the facts before I sent in my report. She perked up a bit, seeming to be relieved that I was at last taking her strange story seriously.

'Miss Cromwell had gone to the lavatory, Mrs Peters is a bit hard of hearing and Miss Macintosh had dived under the table looking for her handkerchief. The voice was in a sort of whisper and a bit hoarse, but it was him all right, there's no doubt about it.' In my mind there was considerable doubt about it.

The doubt lingered and had started to nag, when I thought about Miss Macintosh and her distant cousin who had bequeathed her money to a donkey sanctuary. Misled by Mrs Marsh, the residents had been convinced that the cousin had bequeathed her money to Miss Macintosh. She had gained a good deal of quiet satisfaction in letting them go on thinking it. She had done nothing to set the facts right, except by mentioning the donkey sanctuary to me, and I wouldn't have dreamed of betraying her confidence. I decided to go and see Miss Macintosh and ask her whether she could throw any light on the latest mystery voice at Ivy's seance.

'How was it done?' I asked her after we had touched on the subject without actually saying anything. She gave me the same mischievous look she had given me when she was explaining that she wasn't an heiress but had rather naughtily let Mrs Marsh go on thinking she was. Then she cupped her mouth with her hand and from the corner of the room there came a hoarse penetrating whisper conveying the message that I could expect some good news in the not too distant future. As she and everybody else round the Lodge knew, my third grandchild was due any day. I was less amazed by the message than by the way it was delivered.

'It's a trick I learned a long time ago,' explained Miss Macintosh. 'It used to go down very well at the office parties, especially after we had all had a glass or two of whatever we happened to be drinking. It's quite simple once you get the hang of it.' I never did get the hang of it. However hard I tried my voice still sounded as if it was coming from my mouth rather than from the far corner of the room.

'How did you know about Mrs Peters's son moving to Birmingham?' I asked her, abandoning the attempt at throwing my voice.

'He'd told me himself only that morning,' she said. 'I met him in the market when I was buying a bit of fish for Miss May's lunch and the poor man told me all about it. He said he was dreading telling his mother because although he's nearly fifty she gets very angry if he does anything without getting her permission first.'

I had one more go at being a ventriloquist, then I said I'd have a word with Ivy. Miss Macintosh looked startled but I hastened to assure her that nothing she had said to me would get past her four walls.

I was very tactful with Ivy. I said that maybe it would be better if, instead of holding seances, she stuck to the tea leaves, palms and playing cards. I told her about somebody I once knew who bought a Ouija board and everything was fine until the planchette started moving on its own without any manoeuvring from somebody sitting round the table. The owner of the Ouija board got rid of it at once, terrified of the messages which the moving pencil wrote. The same could happen with her spirit guide. She might never be able to get rid of him unless she made it quite clear that he wasn't wanted. And the only way she could do that was by stopping the seances. She agreed, though a little sadly. She said she could have grown quite fond of him.

Chapter Sixteen

AFTER A LITTLE over a decade of being the matron of the Lodge there were only a few residents left who had been there since I arrived. Miss May was one of them, and surprisingly she had changed very little. Always an invalid, she seemed no more an invalid in her eighties than she had in her seventies. Her rickety legs and angular frame with the bones sticking out everywhere still managed to support the minuscule amount of flesh that covered them. She came over queer no more and no less often than she had always done and spent as much time under the doctor, who had seen her through crisis after crisis. I stayed her with so many nourishing milk puddings, tiny fillets of plaice, the thinnest slices of chicken and mouthfuls of tender steak that I had no fear of her fading away from starvation. She still crocheted shawls, though in simpler patterns after her cataracts started to harden. Her braided hair hadn't whitened and her skin was as unlined as a girl's.

When I heard, after I had left the Lodge, that she had passed peacefully away, I was glad not to have been there when it happened. I had a great fondness for her. I should have missed her warm smile of greeting when she got me up at two in the morning to fill her hot-water bottle. I should have missed the grateful, tear-soaked kisses she showered on me after I had done the dozen or more tasks which she thought of after I had filled the hot-water bottle. Whatever rude things I muttered under my breath as I staggered back to bed when dawn was breaking, I would have been very unhappy if she had drawn her last, fluttering, Horlicks-scented breath while I was with her. I thought when I heard about her death that her ghost must surely haunt the small flatlet where she had lived for so long, as the ghosts of her sisters were said to haunt the old laundry.

Miss Macintosh was still at the Lodge when I left it. She hadn't let age wither her. Her knuckles may have been swollen with rheumatism and her hair snow white but she was still young enough in spirit to take decimal currency, miniskirts and teenagers in her stride. While others round the Lodge were looking shocked and saying how times had changed since they were young, Miss Macintosh was quite prepared to admit that she remembered her mother saying the same when bobbed hair came into fashion. Miss Macintosh had no doubt at all that when today's teenagers were staid old grannies and grand-dads, or bachelor uncles and maiden aunts, they would be saying the same. They would look back nostalgically to the time when they were ripping out seats in the cinema in an excess of emotion stirred up by their favourite pop star and compare those inno-cent pastimes with the terrible things the young would then be doing.

Mrs Turgoose, of course, was still there. Being ninety was something of a feather in her cap. She boasted about it when she had accomplished some small task which she declared would have taxed the strength of somebody half her age and she used it as excuse for not doing something which she could do perfectly well when it suited her. She also put on a year or two when she wanted to make an impression. In less than a month after her ninetieth birthday she had reached the age of ninety-five.

Though she never went out unless she was fetched to a harvest festival supper, a carol concert or a recital given for the elderly, she still managed to start more rumours and spread them further than anybody else. And the rumours had lost none of their inven-tiveness.

'I hear that Mrs Dean's daughter-in-law's gone off with another man,' she said one morning when I was turning her mattress. The mattress was very old and made of feathers. I had to knead it vigorously to get rid of the lumps that had formed throughout the years. But Mrs Turgoose refused to exchange it for one that didn't have to be kneaded. That bed had memories for her, she said, being the one she'd spent her honeymoon on. I knew that was far from the truth. Stew had burnt her original one but she had bought one almost as old through the small ads in the local paper. The thought of sleeping on anything but feathers was more than she could bear. The home help had long since stopped turning her mattress, saying that it took up most of her morning. I put it off as long as I could, by which time it took up most of my morning.

'Where did you hear about Mrs Dean's daughter-in-law?' I asked her, knowing that like the honeymoon bed the story was false. If Mrs Dean's son's wife had left him, his mother was taking it remarkably well. She hadn't mislaid anything since she turned the Lodge upside down looking for a tin opener. She had eventually found it at the bottom of her laundry basket with a number of other things, including a tea cosy which she had accused Stew of taking when he came to hang her curtains up, and a set of spoons for which I got the blame.

'It's common knowledge round here,' replied Mrs Turgoose. 'I first heard it when they took me to that concert at the school where's she's a teacher.'

'What exactly did you hear?' I asked, remembering the innumerable times that Mrs Turgoose had put a different meaning entirely on the things she heard.

'It's not so much what I heard as what I didn't,' she said. 'A nod's as good as a wink to a blind horse and I can take a hint as quick as the next. They didn't have to put it in writing for me to catch on that Mrs Dean's daughter-in-law was going off with one of the men teachers to France. Disgusting, I call it, you expect something better of folks like that.'

'You've got the wrong end of the stick as usual,' I said, giving the mattress an extra thump. 'They haven't gone off together in the way you mean, they're going with other teachers to take a party of children on a camping holiday in France. You could get into a lot of trouble spreading scandal like that.'

'I don't care,' retorted Mrs Turgoose, 'I still think it's a disgrace for a married woman to go to a holiday camp with a man who isn't her husband. Them holiday camps is hotbeds of sin. I went to one once with Gladys Smythe and the man she met at the Labour Party jumble sale. You wouldn't believe the things that went on, and right under our very noses. It was Senior Citizens' week as well. So goodness knows what it's like when there's young ones there.'

I tried not to fall into the mattress at the vision I got of a campful of Senior Citizens sneaking back to their chalets before they were caught by the redcoats and expelled for having orgies.

'Well, never mind about that,' I said sternly. 'All I'm asking is that you think before you say things that could do a great deal of harm.' It was by no means the first time I'd appealed to her better nature and I expected no more response than I'd had in the past.

The rumours about the goings-on at her daughter-in-law's school took a while to reach Mrs Dean's ears. When they did she was as shocked by them as Mrs Turgoose had been.

'I suppose you've heard that the vicar's wife has run off with the headmaster of the school where my daughter-in-law teaches,' she said sadly. 'Poor Mrs Turgoose was heartbroken when she told me. I really can't think what the world's coming to. I thought it was only common people who did things like that.'

As I went on my way I reflected that rumours had always played an important part in the life of the residents, but seldom had anybody been harmed by them. Muddled from the start, they tended to get more muddled as they journeyed along the verandah, unless they were checked sharply by Miss Macintosh who would have no truck with gossip, whether it was true or not. As far as Mrs Turgoose was concerned I knew that when she stopped inventing interesting little stories and passing them on to anybody who would listen, she would have lost her zest for living and I wouldn't have wanted that to happen.

Mrs Peters came to the Lodge after me and left before I did. Her tongue was still sharp and her temper short. She sulked for days when the only home help who had the patience to smile through her tantrums had inconsiderately died while enjoying a well-deserved rest. She sulked even longer when her son's wife brought back her washing which had turned all colours of the rainbow through being bundled into the automatic machine without due regard being paid to the sorting. The downtrodden daughter-in-law suffered the ensuing lashes with fortitude. She knew from experience that if she had brought back the washing exactly as Mrs Peters liked it she would have got no thanks anyway. But there was worse in store for her. She came over to me, wild-eyed and desperate.

'Whatever is to become of us all?' she sobbed brokenly, sinking into my mother's old armchair. 'She's just told me that she wants to leave here and come and live with us. She's got it all planned out. She's going to stay with us and her daughter three months at a time like she did before she moved in here. It was awful then but it'll be a lot worse now. I'm on the change and I get hot flushes and bad heads, and so does her daughter. Can you imagine the bad heads we'll get when she throws one of her tantrums? We shall all be in the psychy ward up at the hospital. All except her, of course.'

I gave the overwrought woman an aspirin and a glass of water and said that I knew how she felt, what with the hot flushes and everything, and she had my sympathy, but as her mother-in-law had set her heart on dividing her remaining years between her family I saw no way of diverting the tragedy.

'She's still quite good on her feet,' I said, thinking I was offering comfort. 'She'll be able to do little things round the house.'

The daughter-in-law helped herself to another aspirin. 'That's what I'm afraid of,' she said. 'She used to do little things round the house before and it caused no end of trouble. She burned holes in all my saucepans and if I said anything she went as white as a sheet and I thought she was going to drop dead on the spot. I was frightened to open my mouth.'

When I said that maybe Mrs Peters had gone as white as a sheet with anger and had no intention of dropping dead on the spot the daughter-in-law said that she had often thought along those lines herself. 'But you can't be too careful with somebody like her. She could do it one day and I'd get the blame.'

I saw Mrs Peters's son in the town after she had removed herself, her little cottage suite and her antique love seat from the Lodge. He looked many years older than when I saw him last. His shoulders were hunched and there was a haunted look in his eyes.

'How is she?' I asked, judging from his appearance that things weren't too good with him.

'She wants to come back to the Lodge,' he said, a flicker of hope temporarily replacing the haunted look. 'She says she can't settle with us. She gets constipated with my wife's cooking and has the runs when she goes to my sister.'

Sorrowfully I had to tell him that there were no vacant flats at the Lodge and even if there were it was unlikely that the charitable body would let her come back as she was obviously in the best of hands and being cared for devotedly by her family. He walked slowly away – a doomed man.

Mrs Peters lived to an overripe old age. I heard that when she died her son took it badly. He had been bound to his mother by such strong ties that he never properly got over the fear of having to make his own decisions. Being a husband and a father had made him no less his mother's son.

The Lodge hadn't changed much over the years. When the fireplaces were ripped out and central heating put in, Stew whitewashed the empty coal cellars, but not everybody was happy at the modern innovation. As Mrs Peters had clung to her mangle, so Miss May clung to her fireplace. After it had gone she sat as far from the radiator as she could get, dreading the moment when steam would belch from the contraption and hit the ceiling with the force of a geyser. She was under the doctor being treated for shock long after the plasterers had filled in the hole where the fireplace had been.

The shower came after the radiators. 'What we need here is a shower,' Ivy said after she came back from Littlehampton, where she had spent a week in one of the hotbeds of sin so roundly condemned by Mrs Turgoose. To everybody's surprise Miss Cromwell went with her. I was shown the holiday snaps. There were several of Ivy paddling with her skirt hitched up, and Miss Cromwell in her gaberdine coat and round hat leaving size ten footprints in the sand. I gathered that though they had never used them there had been showers at Littlehampton.

'Nobody would use it even if we had a shower

installed,' I said, with a pessimism born of long years at the Lodge.

'That's neither here nor there,' said Ivy. 'It would at least look a bit better than that old bath which nobody uses much anyway.'

When the shower was put in, the residents went to have a look at it. A rule was added to the existing ones saying that under no circumstances must a resident avail herself of the new amenity unless the matron was present to supervise the ablutions. I, being fully dressed while I did the supervising, often got as wet as the ladies who decided to take a shower, just to see what it was like. I was glad when the novelty wore off and the residents went back to their old custom of having a good wash down in their living rooms, although it was never as cosy after the fireplaces went.

But if the appearance of the Lodge had changed little since I went there, a marked change had come over the residents. As a result of Ivy's ceaseless endeavours to spread a little happiness, even the most reserved were persuaded to come out of their shell. Instead of sitting behind their net curtains watching what others were doing they went out themselves, strolling along the verandah and having little chats to everybody. Mrs Marsh would have loved it. She would have enjoyed sitting in the porch with Ivy and the others, and having a good gossip with her neighbours instead of trailing round with her empty cup, begging the loan of a bit of sugar in the hope that somebody would ask her in. She would have shambled round to Ivy's place in her slashed-up plimsolls to have her fortune told from the tea leaves, and been as astonished as I was when the forecasting came true.

Chapter Seventeen

THERE ARE MORE ways than one of ending a career that has lasted as long as mine did. I have friends who plodded on until their poor old feet could plod no longer, then they reluctantly stopped being nurses and concentrated on being wives, grannies, or nice old aunts always busily knitting something for somebody. I have other friends who would have plodded on longer than they did if something hadn't happened to bring to a premature end their years of nursing.

I fell somewhere between the two. My poor old feet had been grumbling for a long time about the heavy burden they'd had to carry round from the day I started my training to the day I stopped being the matron of the Lodge. They were in for a long rest when Ivy's interpretation of the things she saw at the bottom of my cup began to take shape.

She had also seen things in my palm that made her shake her head slowly and forebodingly. 'It's the health line,' she said several times after she had scanned all the other lines, including the heart line which had told her a great many things that weren't true. 'There's still that ambulance and you covered in wires,' she said, gazing down at the tea leaves. As far as I could make out the cards also told her some dread thing about my future. Wild horses wouldn't have dragged from her what the dread thing was but she looked gloomy enough to suggest that it could be nothing short of fatal. She was right with the palm and the tea leaf reading but much too pessimistic about the knave of spades, which she said turned up so often that he was giving her the creeps.

The pains in my chest came early one morning when I was plucking up courage to get out of bed and go across to give Miss May her first nourishing meal of the day. I waited for the pains to go, thinking of the cheese I'd had for supper too late the previous evening, but they got worse and worse and worse until they blotted out much of what happened next.

I heard the ambulance men telling me not to worry. I didn't worry. I was too occupied with the pain. And I didn't worry because I was a nurse and knew that I was immune from heart attacks. After all, I had never caught VD when I worked on the VD ward when I was doing my training, and I never caught TB at the sanatorium where the bomb dropped at the start of the war, and I hadn't caught polio or typhoid fever when I was a nurse in those parts of the infectious diseases hospital. The worst I had ever had were the measles, the carbuncles and the minor bit of surgery, none of which had sent an ambulance tearing up the High Street with bells clanging and blue light flashing. Like those who regret that they will be in no condition to enjoy the importance of their own funeral, I felt later that I had missed out on the drama of the matron being removed from the Lodge. I missed out on other things as well.

Though the reception I was given on the ward, with student nurses, a staff nurse, and maybe even a sister waiting to shovel me off the stretcher and into bed, would have gone a long way to satisfy my craving for VIP treatment, I still didn't get a side ward. They, it seemed, were reserved for patients who didn't have to have wires attached.

The first time I opened my eyes and saw my family gathered round the bed three things sprang to my mind: first, amazement at seeing them there, second, a terrible fear that they might be viewing me for the first time without my teeth, and third, the sense of outrage at not being in a side ward. I shut my eyes quickly before the scalding tears of shame rolled down my cheeks.

But after the wires were removed and I had almost forgotten the pains that had taken me into hospital, I lolled back on my pillows and thoroughly enjoyed being a patient. I didn't have a Dole in the bed on my left, but I had a Millie on my right. She also had opened her eyes to find her family gazing at her, she with no teeth and her legs and arms wired to pinging apparatus. We swapped jokes, flouted authority and kept the night nurses awake with our constant call for bedpans. We slandered the sister when she was too far away to hear us, ran down the nurses and argued with the doctors. But we ate our steamed fish and yoghurt obediently.

Not once did either of us get up at the crack of dawn to push the tea trolley round the ward. For, as Millie said, 'We might as well make the most of it while we're here, there'll be nobody to give us cups of tea when we get home.' Like me she had grown used to drinking her morning tea with only the paper for company.

Having a heart attack isn't the best way of changing one's life style, it is too often the means by which a life is ended or permanently disabled, but I was one of the lucky ones. After months of slow recovery, hindered maybe by the knowledge that my nursing days were over, I borrowed a typewriter, bought a ream of paper and started my first book. Putting the memories down on paper with two fingers crashing at the keys was occupational therapy which gave me fresh hope, something to get up for in the morning, and more than enough to fill the idle hours. Finally there was the earth-shaking letter from a publisher saying that he'd accepted the book.

I have much to be thankful for.

About the Author

Brought up in Lincolnshire, Evelyn Prentis left home at eighteen to become a nurse. She later moved to London during the war, where she married and raised her family. Like so many other nurses, she went back to hospital and used any spare time she might have had bringing up her children and running her home. Born in 1915, she sadly died in 2001 at the age of eighty-five.

Evelyn published five books about her life as a nurse, and Ebury Press have reissued them all. *A Nurse in Time*, *A Nurse in Action*, *A Nurse and Mother* and *Matron at Last* are all available and *Matron in Charge* now completes the series.

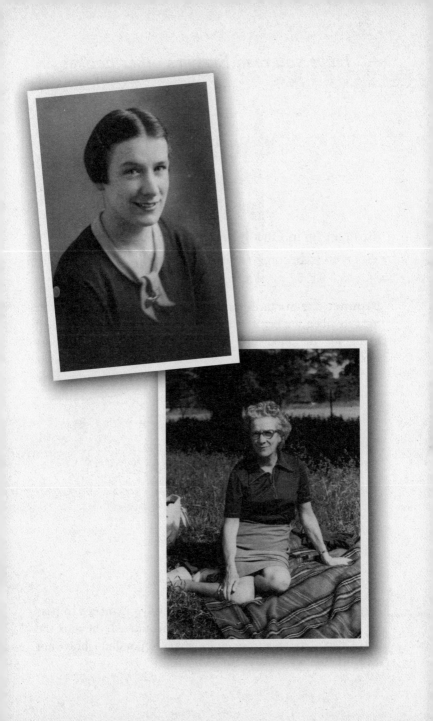

Have you read Evelyn's other books?

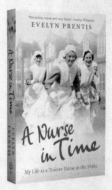

Desperate circumstances were something Evelyn had to get very used to when she began her life as a nurse. In 1934 Evelyn left home for the first time to enrol as a trainee at a busy Nottingham hospital and *A Nurse in Time* is her affectionate and funny account of those days of dedication, hardship and joy.

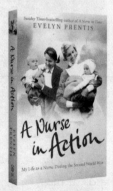

Surprising Matron as well as herself, Evelyn managed to pass her Finals and become a staff-nurse. Encouraged, she took the brave leap of moving from Nottingham to London – brave not least because war was about to break…

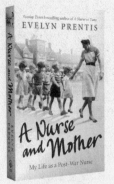

At the end of the Second World War, as husbands came back to Civvy Street their wives had the luxury of staying at home with the children. But soon Evelyn realised she had to find part-time work to make ends meet, and to her astonishment she was offered part-time hours at her old hospital.

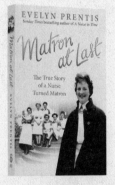

After working as a nurse for thirty years, Evelyn left the hospital to become a full-time matron at the Lodge – a home for elderly ladies of reduced circumstances. Even though it did mean she was on call twenty-four hours a day, this is Evelyn's funny and affectionate memoir of her years – at last! – as a matron.

www.eburypublishing.co.uk